Senior Years

Senior Years

Understanding Your Dog's Aging Process

John K. Hampton, Jr., Ph.D.
and
Suzanne H. Hampton, Ph.D.

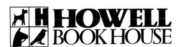
HOWELL BOOK HOUSE

New York

Maxwell Macmillan Canada
Toronto

Maxwell Macmillan International
New York   Oxford   Singapore   Sydney

Howell Book House   Maxwell Macmillan Canada, Inc.
Macmillan Publishing Company   1200 Eglinton Avenue East
866 Third Avenue   Suite 200
New York, NY 10022   Don Mills, Ontario M3C 3N1

Macmillan Publishing Company is part of the Maxwell Communication Group of Companies.

Library of Congress Cataloging-in-Publication Data

Hampton, John K.
   Senior years: understanding your dog's aging process / John K.
Hampton, Jr., and Suzanne H. Hampton.
      p.   cm.
   Includes index.
   ISBN 0-87605-734-2
   1. Dogs—Aging. 2. Dogs—Diseases. 3. Dogs—Health.
   4. Veterinary geriatrics. I. Hampton, Suzanne H. II. Title.
   SF768.2.D6H36 1993
   636.7′089897—dc20   92–14584
                                                                  CIP

Macmillan books are available at special discounts for bulk purchases for sales promotions, premiums, fund-raising, or educational use. For details, contact:

Special Sales Director
Macmillan Publishing Company
866 Third Avenue
New York, NY 10022

10 9 8 7 6 5 4 3 2 1
Printed in the United States of America

To Champion Limebell Roaring Forties.
She grew old—and venerable.

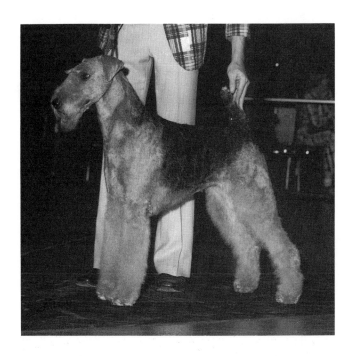

Contents

Acknowledgments

Many books benefit by having someone critically read early versions; Joyce Murphy is thanked for that valuable contribution.

The talents of Joanna Tommasacci are reflected in many of the drawings.

Finally, special thanks are extended to Marcy L. Zingler, our editor at Howell, for an amazing degree of patience and perseverance; her efforts made a significant contribution to clarity.

Preface

SCIENTIFIC TERMINOLOGY is sometimes used in this book, but an attempt has been made to prevent it from being burdensome. However, it is justified at times to prepare a reader to seek further information in the library or elsewhere by knowing appropriate terms. Some readers will be accustomed to speaking of a male dog as a *dog* and denoting a female as a *bitch*. However, to accommodate those not familiar with these terms, *dog* is used generically and does not refer to the sex of an animal. *Male* or *female* is used when needed to indicate the sex, although the term *bitch* is occasionally used for a female.

Boldface type is used for technical terms that may be unfamiliar. However, they are only boldfaced the first time they appear in a chapter. Parentheses enclose alternative terms or provide clarification of terms. Material is often repeated in separate chapters whenever that helps explain an issue and to save the reader the effort of locating supporting information in other places. Cross references to other chapters are used to indicate that other or more complete information on a subject is available. Sidebars, illustrations, and tables are used to amplify unfamiliar or difficult subjects. Material in these forms is not essential to reasonable understanding of the discussions in regular text, but they will often help clarify concepts or present a concise collection of facts.

Because the topic of this book is the elderly dog and its ailments, no attempt has been made to treat all knowledge of physiology—just the subjects that provide background for understanding the aging phenomena. Biomedical knowledge has been acquired from study of dogs and humans independently. Many "facts" have been shown to be common to both, and it is reasonable to assume that they are in other cases. Therefore, human values have sometimes been used when it is believed that they probably do not differ from the dog. For example, human data have been used to discuss effects of exercise because much more detailed measurements have been made in humans.

It is not always correct to ascribe certain information to *all* dogs. The selective breeding that produced the many dog breeds has, inevitably, sorted genes that relate to features other than size, behavior, and appearance. Consequently, various *invisible* traits make some dogs considerably different from others. Whenever breed traits have been found, they are reported in this book. Further study may modify such information, and your veterinarian's experiences may indicate other important variations.

In many places, typical therapies for diseases are mentioned. This may help the reader anticipate the nature of some treatments; it certainly is not meant to encourage the reader to attempt treatments independent of a veterinarian's attention.

1

Introduction: An Overview of Aging and Its Understanding

$\mathbf{B}$ECAUSE YOU ARE INTERESTED in aging dogs, we feel you will want to gain a broad overview of the phenomenon of aging, as well as information about specific ailments. This chapter is important in that it provides an overview of several topics highly relevant to aging. Read it as a survey of several important biological principles, as well as for a preview of what is to come later.

Throughout this book we will emphasize the role of physiology, a part of biology that deals with function, because aging is best understood in the light of the changes in function that accompany aging.

STRUCTURE AND PHYSIOLOGY

Because physiology is the study of the mechanisms fundamental to life, looking at the aging dog as a physiologist does will enhance your understanding of bodily functions and will provide insights beyond the simple observations of cause and effect.

Because the dog is a large multicellular animal, there are challenging functional (physiological) requirements based on cellular relationships. Therefore, you should understand the **anatomical** organization of an individual animal. The smallest individual unit of life that can survive alone is the **cell**. There are many different types of cells, all of which come from an original cell created by the union of a **spermatozoan** (sperm) and an **ovum** (egg). A **tissue** is a mass of cells having similar characteristics. **Organs** (e.g., heart, stomach, brain) consist of specific tissues that collectively perform certain functions dependent upon cell and tissue associations. Two or more organs often work together in an **organ system**.

Tissues also contain important **cell products** such as the large chemical molecules **collagen** and **elastin**, which provide mechanical properties. Nerves, blood, and blood vessels are integrated within all organs.

You can easily see how alterations in the function of the cells of one tissue can have serious consequences on how that tissue functions in an organ or organ system. Aging seems to be characterized by an accumulation of such failures and the widespread effects they cause.

COMMUNICATION BETWEEN CELLS

Two great organ systems provide much of the communication between functional units of the body, as seen in Table 1.1. The nervous system acts to control movement and is the source of that remarkable characteristic called intelligence. It also makes it possible for the organism to be aware of and react with its environment. More chemical in nature, the endocrine system uses communication hormones as **messengers** to affect the function of a great array of other organs and tissues. Also, special forms of communication exist within the body's immune system, as you will see in a later chapter.

TABLE 1.1   Body Systems and Major Functions

Regulatory
  Nervous System
  Endocrine System
Nutritional
  Intake
    Gastrointestinal System
  Assimilation
    Nutrition
    Metabolism
Excretory
  Renal (Kidney) System
  Respiratory (Pulmonary) System
Distributive
  Cardiovascular System
  Blood and Body Fluids
Protective
  Immune System
  Integumentary (Skin) System
Reproductive
  Reproductive System

2

AGING AND EVOLUTION

Evolution provides a concept of the relationships between many different forms of living things, including their physiology. It is well established that organisms can be changed by selectively controlling their reproduction. This is dramatically evidenced by the many breeds of dogs that have been produced. The evolution of physiological and biochemical systems helps the physiologist recognize how certain functions have reached their current forms.

A KEY CONCEPT IN AGING—HOMEOSTASIS

Perhaps the most important concept in physiology is **homeostasis**. This concept refers to the way in which the body maintains internal stability by regulating its internal functions. A constant and appropriate environment must be provided to each of the millions of cells found in the body.

Ideas derived from views of evolution can be applied to the concept of homeostasis. When primitive cells were in their most favorable environment (i.e., a large, unchanging ocean mass), they prospered. Complex organisms, such as dogs, must also have mechanisms that maintain an ideal environment for each cell. The immediate environment of all cells in large animals is provided by close contact with the smallest blood vessels, the capillaries.

It has been said that blood and body fluids should be viewed as "the sea within us." The roles of the lungs, kidneys, and gastrointestinal system serve to keep the blood's composition constant in order to meet all the cells' environmental, nutritional, and excretory needs. In other words, to maintain homeostasis it is necessary to maintain an ideal environment around each cell.

STRESS AND HOMEOSTASIS

The term *stress* has been used so carelessly that its meaning is now vague. It is common to say that challenge produces stress. That is not necessarily so; challenges may serve as beneficial stimuli. Appropriate exercise may stimulate muscles to grow and adapt; excessive exercise may destroy muscle cells and disrupt muscle metabolism. Stress exists when conditions threaten to change the healthy organism unless the organism makes changes that will maintain homeostasis. It is known that sufficient threat brings about an outpouring of certain hormones and activation of certain nervous system functions. These can temporarily help an animal survive in spite of the unstable state (loss of homeostasis) that occurs. Of course, if these responses to stress are insufficient or if the stress lasts too long, homeostasis does not last and the individual animal experiences the loss of homeostasis as degraded cell function.

We see stress effects more easily in the very young and the very old. Your older dog no longer has the functional ability to respond to threat (cold weather,

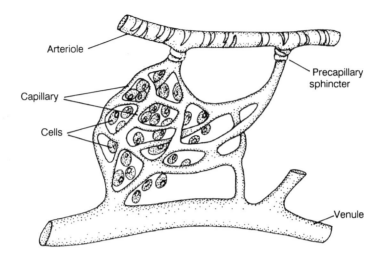

Arteriole

Precapillary
sphincter

Capillary

Cells

Venule

Relationship Between Capillaries and Cells   This illustration shows the intimate relationship between cells of the body and capillaries, the smallest blood vessels. The fluids that surround cells provide an environment that has a composition similar to blood. If the blood composition is kept normal and constant, cells exist in an ideal environment.

an ingested poison, boarding in a strange kennel, anesthesia) as would a healthy younger dog. Even stimuli that are slight can be stressful because of the loss of ability to adapt.

PHYSIOLOGICAL CONTROL

Control systems exist so that order will be maintained within the body. One of these systems is known as the **feedback** system, where a function is modified by an end product of that function. For example, a hormone, meant to affect some distant target cells, may also act upon the cells that produced the hormone, therefore reducing its own further production.

This feedback is not a matter of off-and-on control that works as a switch might. The control is relative to the activity; that is, a little product inhibits slightly and a large amount inhibits greatly. This is an example of **negative feedback**. Although quite uncommon, **positive feedback** systems also exist. For example, when, during the birth process, uterine contractions push a puppy's head against the opening of the womb, that pressure stimulates further uterine contractions.

Another system might be called a **check-and-balance** arrangement. The **autonomic** portion of the nervous system provides an example. Two different components of the autonomic nervous system often connect to the same organ or tissue with one of the divisions being inhibitory and the other stimulative. The target tissue responds to the averaged effect of the two. For example, heart rate is increased by **sympathetic** nervous activity and slowed by the **parasympathetic** division. In this way, heart rate is under dual influence and will reflect the balance of the two components. Two hormones, **insulin** and **glucagon**, have such a relationship in regulating blood sugar. This is a finely tuned control mechanism.

BIOLOGICAL CLOCKS

Some patterns of function (e.g., sleeping at intervals) persist even when your dog is removed from any stimuli that would give information about the time of day because they are innate cycles. One timed biological event is the onset of **puberty**. This happens to all healthy dogs and happens within a rather narrow range of ages.

For a long time, biologists have known that many animals follow patterns of life based on a daily (**circadian**) cycle. It is a common view that some mechanism recognizes and tallies this daily interval and uses this information to turn on the functions that bring about the changes of puberty. The **menopause** of human females also falls into this category.

Are some of the changes that accompany aging, including death, similarly programmed by **biological clocks**? This idea of biological clocks and how they may be set suggests that some of life's events are programmed, a consideration of great importance to a study of aging.

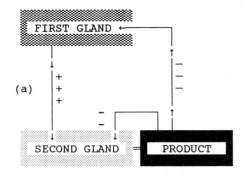

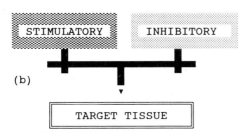

Control Systems Principles The most common mechanism controlling body physiology is a feedback loop where an end effect of the function affects the function itself. Usually, this is a negative feedback system, as in (a). In other cases (b), the effect may be both stimulatory and inhibitory, with the end result being the weighted strength of the two.

LONGEVITY

Demographers provide information about the **average (mean) life expectancy**, **maximum life span**, and **survivorship curves** of animal **species**.

A graph of numbers of survivors in a population over time is a survivorship curve. As causes of death are conquered, the graph will show the pattern of death due to a failure of homeostasis rather than traditional diseases. After removal of deaths attributable to random disease and accidents, the graph's curve will show deaths within a narrower range of ages, and the ages are nearer the fixed point of maximum life span. Thus, modern veterinary medicine and healthy life-styles have affected mean life expectancy but not maximal life span of the domestic dog.

Some procedures do extend maximum life span in experiments with some animals. Slight in their effect, they are impractical to apply to humans or dogs. An exception is the remarkable result of caloric restriction in animals on otherwise sound diets. A later chapter deals with this subject.

VARIABILITY AMONG DOG BREEDS AND THE AGED

A most noticeable feature of an aged animal population is the **range** (i.e., variability) of function seen in any given age group. At any given older age, individuals near death because of many systems failing to maintain homeostasis may be contrasted with those who may expect many more years of good health. This variability is not trivial to the understanding of age changes. For example, older dogs may well have nutritional needs and metabolic characteristics that are different and more limiting than when they were young. We must look at the aged as a population in which some of the physiological characteristics of the young continue, but in which other characteristics become altered in an irregular way.

Because each breed of dogs has its own characteristic maximum life span, it is important to compare individuals only within a breed. Not only are breeds different in size, each breed is the result of selective (intentional or unintentional) breeding. Because appearance or temperament was the goal of selective breeding, many physiological characteristics have been selected without our knowledge. Current veterinary practice acknowledges these functional differences when they are known.

BODY SIZE—ITS SIGNIFICANCE

Not only are breeds different from each other in certain ways, but the size differences of members within a breed is important—and the extreme size differences between breeds must be taken into account. Older dogs require attention to these differences more than do younger ones.

A primary concern is the dosage of medicine or the ingestion of poisons. In most cases, the effect of a substance is based on the speed of its excretion or metabolic change into something else. Liver and kidney functions are commonly involved. The point to consider is not just size based on weight, but the **metabolic rate** (the rate of chemical reactions) of the individual animal. One way to estimate the metabolic rate is to consider the animal's whole body surface area, which has been shown to be proportional to its metabolic rate. Thus, a dog of one pound will have much more surface area per pound than will a one-hundred-pound dog. If proper dosage for a Great Dane is administered to a Boston Terrier on the basis of weight, it may well be inadequate. On the other hand, proper dosage for the Boston Terrier multiplied by the weight factor and given to a Great Dane might be a serious overdose.

In the case of some substances, this principle may be overlooked or only invite caution when the animals are young and have considerable ability to maintain homeostasis. The older dog may be seriously handicapped by either an underdose of medicine which does not serve its purpose, or an *overdose*, which is *toxic*. These principles are discussed in the chapter Drugs, Anesthesia, and Surgery in the Aging Dog.

AGING—A DEFINITION

Aging is the accumulation of negative changes in physiology that occur from the time of conception until death. But *all changes* between conception and death *are not the aging process.* Aging should be associated only with those alterations in functional capacity that make the organism less able to maintain homeostasis. Such changes accumulate and reach a point when a vital state cannot be maintained and life cannot continue. The causes and mechanisms of these changes should be known for a full understanding of aging.

Various breeds of dogs are known to have characteristic life spans. In general, larger breeds live shorter lives. The opinion varies, but it seems reasonable to consider larger breeds "old" starting at about five years of age. Smaller breeds seem to reach the same stage of life around seven years or so. One source suggests that of the over 50 million dogs in this country, the number that are over six years old approaches 50 percent.

AGING—DOES IT HAVE A PURPOSE?

Does aging have a purpose? This question must be addressed by all who are interested in aging. The aging and dying of complex organisms is universal and does not prevent species survival. Therefore, does it enhance species survival?

Sexual reproduction has been seen as the cardinal element for the survival of a species. Many inherited features exist in each individual and these attributes are the bases of abilities to survive in the available environment. In nature, environments change from time to time. *A species has a greater chance to survive when composed of members that vary.* This varied composition makes it probable that some individuals will maintain homeostasis in the face of a moderately threatening environmental change because they have a more suitable genetic makeup. If all members of a species were genetically identical, all would have the same chance of survival—and nonsurvival. Reproduction by sexual means causes continuous sorting of the gene pool, increasing the chance that even more suitable individuals may emerge in the population. Reproduction provides an adaptive mechanism for species survival just as individual death might avoid overcrowding. Making room for genetically suitable individuals appears to some as a reason for aging and death.

Other authorities do not feel that the "living space" idea is valid. Wild animals, as well as humans and domestic animals, have died from various causes that prevented any significant number from reaching maximum life span. Indeed, human mean life expectancy is still quite low in much of the world, and this is so for dogs in the wild. Thus, the balance between death and reproduction almost always has provided as much opportunity for space and genetic renewal as aging-based death might provide.

2

Animal Cells: Structure, Function, and Cancer-Producing Genetic Errors

---

THE MILLIONS OF CELLS of a dog's body that are not involved in sexual reproduction are referred to as **somatic** cells. There are many different kinds of cells, each type with its own specialized function, yet each cell has virtually the same complement of genetic material. Because of this, each cell begins with the potential to become one of many different types of cells. However, during development, specific portions of the genetic material within each cell are inactivated, with the remaining active genes governing the cell's characteristic functions.

In order to perform unique functions, some cells specialize to such an extent that they can no longer divide for the purpose of replacing lost cells (e.g., neurons and skeletal muscle cells). However, other cells (e.g., epithelial cells) are able to divide rapidly and often; it is these cells that are most susceptible to becoming cancerous.

It appears that cancer cells may be those cells that have actually regressed so that inactive genes are "turned on" and begin to function again. Recent studies have shown that the aberrant functioning of certain genes (referred to as

oncogenes) are responsible for the uncontrolled growth of some cancer cells. These genes behave as agents for growth-stimulating factors, unlike normal genes that are ordinarily subjected to control mechanisms.

Cancer, then, is the uncontrolled growth of a group of cells. Intensive study and heroic treatment efforts have provided notable cure rates for only a few kinds of cancer. Nonetheless, the knowledge gained to date has had broad usefulness. The process that produces a malignant cell's uncontrolled multiplication may involve the same or similar genetic mechanisms as those that cause cells to stop dividing and functioning properly as aging occurs.

Studies of cells in tissue culture in the laboratory have materially added to our knowledge of them. Certain aspects of aging theory have come from the observation that many cells seem to have a fundamentally limited life span **in vitro** (in tissue culture systems) and **in vivo** (in the living animal).

THE ORIGIN OF CELL TYPES

Coded **genetic material**, DNA, exists in both **germinal** cells (stem cells for sperm and ova) and **somatic** cells (all nongerminal cells) in a state of paired **chromosomes**. When ova (eggs) are produced in the female, the DNA in each ovum divides so that each ovum will have only one chromosome from each pair. This special type of cell division is called **meiosis**. Because sperm (spermatozoa) are similarly produced, a spermatozoan's contribution to a fertilized egg will complement the genes and chromosomes in the ovum, making a cell that is once again genetically complete. From this single cell, all the types of somatic cells in the new individual develop by a process called **differentiation**. Differentiation consists of a series of divisions in which complete copies of DNA-containing chromosomes are incorporated into each daughter cell. This is called **mitotic** division.

After the fertilized egg cell divides several times, the daughter cells, and perhaps their environment, release signals that cause each cell's genetic information to be expressed. According to the stimulus they receive, cells begin differentiating into one of the three basic types of embryonic tissue layers from which all cell types arise. These embryonic layers are called **ectoderm, meso-derm**, and **endoderm**.

Throughout the process of tissue differentiation (**histogenesis**), the genetic materials within each cell guide that cell's development, as well as controlling the function of the fully differentiated cell. In cancer, the opposite appears to occur; cells undergo **dedifferentiation** and lose prior restrictions.

ANATOMY OF THE CELL

A cell (see accompanying illustration) is encompassed by a **plasma membrane (cell membrane)** that is **lipoidal** (fatty) in nature. This fact is significant

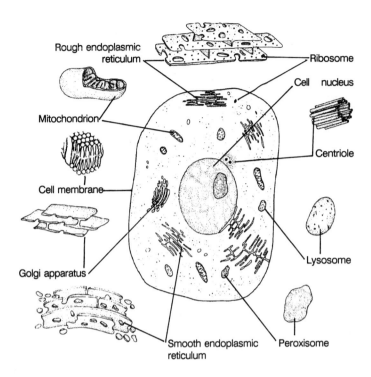

Rough endoplasmic reticulum

Ribosome

Cell nucleus

Mitochondrion

Centriole

Cell membrane

Golgi apparatus

Lysosome

Smooth endoplasmic reticulum

Peroxisome

Anatomy of a Cell Cells contain a variety of miniature organs (organelles), each having unique functions. See the text and Table 2.1 for further information about the structures illustrated in this diagram.

because the environment within and outside of the membrane consists of water and substances that are dissolved in water.

The passage of **solutes** and water through cell membranes is provided for by special molecules of protein and carbohydrate that are built into the membranes. These **membrane inclusions** not only aid transport, but some also serve to identify the cell to the immune system, enabling it to recognize foreign or abnormal cells. Other membrane inclusions are quite important because they provide binding sites for agents, such as hormones, that bring specific stimuli to cells.

These proteins are part of normal cell membranes and serve as binding sites for hormones and other specifically bound substances. They are sometimes reduced in number during aging. For example, insulin binding sites on cell membranes are reduced in Type II diabetes.

Within the cell, the cell **nucleus** is also surrounded by a membrane (the **nuclear envelope**) but it is unlike the plasma membrane that surrounds a cell. Fairly large molecules pass through pores in the nuclear envelope. Coded information in the nuclear DNA (in the form of genes) is **transcribed** into smaller molecules of RNA that then cross the nuclear membrane. RNA molecules act within the cytoplasm to **translate** this information by the production of highly specific protein molecules.

Most of the cell's "machinery" is located outside the nucleus in the **cytosol**, the liquid phase within the cell. The structures that comprise this intracellular machinery are little organs termed **organelles**. Some important organelles are listed in Table 2.1, along with the primary functions of each.

SPECIAL CELLS

Some cells undergo such extensive specialization that they develop unusual properties that are worth noting. Such a cell is the nerve cell, called a **neuron**. The shape and size of neurons are elaborate, and within a single neuron different parts have specific functions—each part could almost be called a microorgan. Because of this extreme degree of specialization, the neuron cannot divide as most cells can. Unless current research in this area reveals new principles, replacing lost neurons appears impossible.

Muscle cells, like neurons, can transmit a special form of electrical activity over their membranes and, like neurons, are referred to as **excitable tissues**. Skeletal muscle cells (fibers) also have specialized to such an extent that one unit is actually several cells fused together, sharing several nuclei. These cells cannot divide to increase the number of cells—growth takes place by enlarging existing cells. Cardiac (heart) muscle has this characteristic. Smooth muscle cells can multiply.

The body contains two types of glands that secrete special products. Cells of **exocrine glands** produce substances that are passed by tubes or ducts to another area. Examples are sweat glands; glands in the liver, pancreas, and intestinal wall that produce digestive substances; and salivary glands. **Endocrine glands** have no ducts, but produce hormones that go directly into the blood for

TABLE 2.1   Intracellular Organelles and Their Functions

Ribosomes—Guided by genetic instructions, these are the sites of protein synthesis.

Mitochondria—Microstructures that contain the myriad of enzymes that direct production of energy from food.

Lysosomes—Microstructures filled with powerful enzymes capable of digesting many substances, including bacteria.

Peroxisomes—Also containing enzymes, but mainly oxidase types capable of acting on hydrogen peroxide and other oxidizable material such as alcohols and phenols.

Microtubules—Support cell structure and provide channels to move substances from one part of the cell to another.

Microfilaments—Involved in muscle cell contraction; provide cell structure in other cells with help from the microtubules.

Centrioles—Participate in and help organize the process of cell division.

Golgi apparatus—Helps form condensed protein units for secretion; involved in fat and carbohydrate metabolism; forms lysosomes.

transport to sites of action. Endocrine glands constitute the major chemical control system for the body and are discussed in detail in the chapter The Endocrine System.

Mature red blood cells (RBCs) of mammals are remarkable because they have no nucleus and, therefore, lack the functional DNA of other cells. RBC nuclei are lost during extensive differentiation (specialization) from more primitive cells (**stem cells**) located in the bone marrow. The RBC has a life span of about 120 days in the human and 90 to 135 days in the dog. The age of each RBC is recognized by the spleen and other specialized cells, and results in the removal and destruction of old RBCs.

CANCER—DIAGNOSIS AND TREATMENT

Cancer growths (**malignant neoplasms**) refer to disease conditions that result from genetically altered cells. The type of cells involved determines the term used to describe the cancer. If epithelium is the cell type affected, it is called a **carcinoma**. An **adenocarcinoma** is derived from gland cells (*adeno* means gland). **Sarcomas** are cancer growths of the connective tissues, more specifically designated as **fibrosarcoma** (of fibrous tissue), **osteosarcoma** (of bone tissue), and **chondrosarcoma** (of cartilage). Somewhat differently named, **glial** cells, which are nonnerve cells of the central nervous system, give rise to **gliomas**. Bone marrow cells are the origin of **myelomas** and **leukemia**.

Cancer has at least two phases in its development. First, it must be *initiated* by some stimulus or agent acting on a cell, which then gives rise to a group of identical, abnormal cells (a **clone**). The molecular changes that initiate the first stage of development of the cancer growth always seem to involve the DNA within the nucleus. Only cells capable of mitosis (dividing) can undergo this **neoplastic transformation**; cardiac and skeletal muscle, red blood cells, and neurons (nerve cells) ordinarily cannot do so.

A second influence must come from a **promoter** in order for cells to make the full transition to cancer cells. Once the transition has been accomplished, uncontrolled cell growth is characteristic. Cancer cells, unlike normal cells, may be grown virtually indefinitely in tissue culture. Also, such cells may relocate to different parts of the body (**metastasis**). Aggressive invasion of healthy tissue is common, thus the name *cancer* ("the crab").

In addition to **neoplasia** (new growth), another characteristic of cancer is **anaplasia**. This is a condition that disrupts the normal biochemical orderliness and the structural orderliness of a tissue's cells. The inhibiting effect of cell-to-cell contact is lost in cancerous tissues so that cells multiply into large, overlapping masses.

Familiar initiators and/or promoters (i.e., **carcinogens**) come from ionizing radiation (X rays, gamma rays, etc.), some viruses, and environmental pollutants (certain insecticides, food dyes, etc.). Less familiar is the fact that some products of normal metabolism and substances in ordinary, healthy foodstuff also have the potential to modify DNA.

Chemical carcinogens account for about 80 percent of malignant neoplasms (cancers). Most chemicals associated with cancer are actually processed in the liver and converted to highly reactive molecules. A major function of the liver is to "detoxify" substances, but in some cases the outcome is not completely desirable.

During embryonic development, cells from the thymus gland learn to identify certain genetically determined surface characteristics of normal cells as "self." Later, cells from the thymus gland recognize as "nonself" the body cells that have become cancer cells or have been introduced from the outside (organ transplants), and mount an attack against them. These cells of the **immune surveillance system** also continuously destroy many other cells that are in the process of differentiating into malignant forms.

The immune response becomes depressed in dogs with cancer. Recent study has cast light on this in two areas. In one case, researchers have shown that a specific **lymphokine** (a substance from certain immune cells), which ordinarily attracts immune cells to foreign cells, is not produced in sufficient quantity. The other defect is an inappropriate activation of some immune cells (**suppressor T lymphocytes**), whose function is to turn off immune activity when it is no longer needed. Thus, the desired attack on abnormal cells is aborted too soon. This will be addressed again in the chapter The Protective Role of the Immune System.

Cancer is now better understood because of the discovery of oncogenes. These are specific genes that can transform normal cells into malignant ones—*onco* refers to cancer. Certain normal genes that can become oncogenes (**proto-oncogenes**) initiate production of growth-promoting factors that are needed when cells multiply for normal cell replacement or wound healing. These genes (many have been identified) normally are under controls that limit their activity. However, if they become relocated within DNA, or if some alteration in closely associated DNA removes their controls, they produce growth factors continuously, and stimulate the unregulated growth of malignant neoplasia. Indeed, carcinogens that act as cancer promoters may specifically act to free oncogenes from their normal controls.

A single, activated oncogene is apparently not sufficient to bring about the uncontrolled growth of cancer cells. In some cases, two oncogenes acting together may do so—as appears to happen with the oncogenes called **ras** and **myc.** The normal *ras* proto-oncogene codes for a small protein that is thought to indirectly govern cell growth. The protein coded by the *myc* proto-oncogene binds to DNA and may affect or regulate DNA transcription.

Both the *ras* and *myc* oncogenes are associated with an acute form of human leukemia known as Burkitt's lymphoma. It is likely that malignant lymphoma, the most common cancer of the blood-cell-producing system in dogs (with a significantly high incidence in Boxers, Labrador Retrievers, and Scottish Terriers), arises by a similar mechanism.

However, it is important to note, although our knowledge of oncogenes may be interesting and useful, there are many types of cancer for which there is no evidence of oncogene involvement.

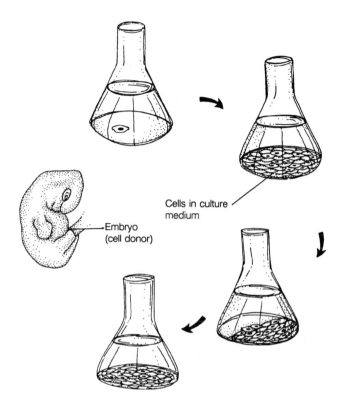

Cell Growth in Tissue Culture Normal embryonic tissue cells grown in a flask in a nutrient solution multiply until they cover the bottom, stopping as a result of increased contact with one another. If the cell mass is divided and fresh nutrient is supplied, the cells double in number before stopping again. After many such "doublings," growth becomes slowed and finally stops entirely. When cells are taken from older donors, there are fewer doublings.

Many cancers respond poorly to **chemotherapy**, and drug resistance seems to be an inherent property of tumor cells. The mechanisms involved are related to the very same systems that help protect against DNA damage or affect DNA repair. Chemotherapy, when directed toward killing cancer cells by blocking DNA function, actually stimulates cells to amplify their defenses against the drugs. This underscores the current cancer therapy research oriented toward building the immune system.

Cancer As It Relates to Aging

Study of cancer is most relevant to the study of aging. Not only is the incidence of cancer markedly increased as dogs age, but the study of the causes of cancer promises to make its role in aging clearer. Especially attractive is the idea that oncogenes, rather than being released from suppression, may be more

Labels within figure:
Cells in culture medium
Embryo (cell donor)

rigidly suppressed or lost in the course of time, bringing about many of the features of aging such as tissue wasting and slow wound repair.

Tissue Culture Studies

A great deal of information about cancer has been obtained from cells maintained in **tissue culture**. During the 1950s, scientists at the Wistar Institute, Leonard Hayflick and Paul Moorhead, examined the possibility that cancer cell cultures might transmit a cancer-causing virus to normal cells in tissue culture. At that time, many transformed cells had been cultured successfully. All those cells that could exist indefinitely in tissue culture shared substantial characteristics with cancer cells. Subsequent research showed that cells that did not transform had limited lives in culture. This line of research showed that healthy cells from mammal embryos (e.g., lung fibroblasts) would divide in culture until they covered the bottom of the culture vessel. They would then cease growing because of **contact inhibition**, a physical interaction of cells that restricts cell

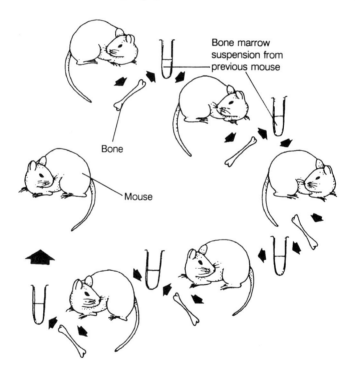

The Effects of Host on Cell Life Span   Mice exposed to sufficient ionizing radiation to destroy their bone marrow (the source of their blood cells) may serve as hosts for bone marrow transfusions from younger animals of the same genetic strain. Repopulated with blood-forming cells, these mice may donate their new marrow to another irradiated host. In this way, use of serial hosts demonstrates that the original cells can live longer than the original donor.

division. If half of these cells were removed, they would grow to cover the bottom of the flask again. After a number of doublings, further growth ceased.

Tissue Transplants

It has been found that such cultured cells had a number of doublings inversely related to the age of their donor. Several reports have confirmed this phenomenon when cells from human embryos and from humans up to their early nineties were used. Experiments in laboratory animals have shown that the survival of a skin transplant, for example, was a function of the age of the donor, not the recipient.

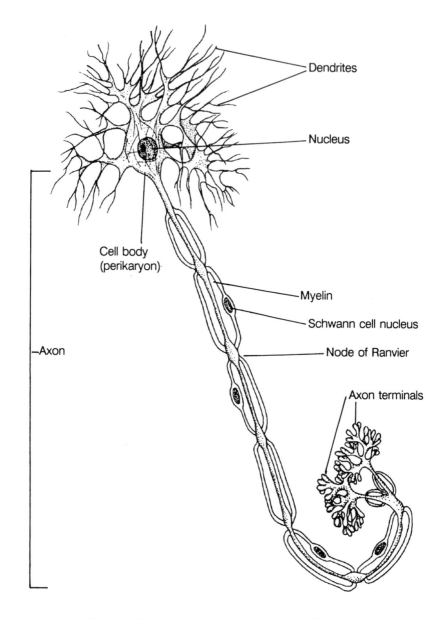

Dendrites

Nucleus

Cell body
(perikaryon)

Myelin

Schwann cell nucleus

–Axon

Node of Ranvier

Axon terminals

Anatomy of a Neuron   Neurons vary widely in their anatomy. However, the basic form is illustrated here, showing the four main portions. The number of contact sites on dendrites and axonal knobs may be far greater than illustrated. Schwann cells wrap the axon at intervals with myelin, an electrical insulator.

3

The Excitable Tissues:
Nerve and Muscle Cells

NERVE CELLS and cells of muscle are excitable. An "electrical charge" exists across the membranes that surround these cells. If altered by suitable stimuli, this change can then be propagated along the membrane. This constitutes the conduction of an impulse.

In order to accommodate their specialized functions, nerve cells, as well as skeletal and cardiac muscle cells, have differentiated considerably from the cells of their origin. Because of this superspecialization, the ability to grow or repair by cell division is lost.

Since they cannot further divide, the body provides the protection of the skull and spinal vertebrae to the cells of the **central nervous system** (CNS), which number many trillion. Despite this physical protection, *nerve cells are lost as aging occurs*. However, some have the ability to reorient connections between themselves within the nervous system. This considerably offsets the reduction in function that would be expected to occur.

Skeletal and cardiac muscle cells are not so well protected; when one is lost, it is not replaced. However, these muscle cells can grow in size individually. Although this allows some degree of compensation, *muscle mass is characteristically lost during aging*.

PRIMARY NERVE CELLS (NEURONS) AND OTHER NERVE CELLS (NEUROGLIA): FUNCTION AND STRUCTURE

Neurons

Nerve cells, usually called **neurons**, have elaborate shapes and size variations. Starting as much simpler cells, the development of neurons is stimulated and guided by small proteins known as **nerve growth factors** (NGF). As they develop into neurons, they lose the ability to divide; so growth and repair of nervous structures is lost.

A mature neuron contains its genetic material (DNA) within the nucleus of the cell body area. Projections at one end of the neuron are called **dendrites**. These are treelike and sometimes have thousands of branches. The **axon** is a single projection from the cell body that ends in numerous branches. These branches have unique **axon terminals** (sometimes called **terminal knobs**).

How Neurons Transmit Diseases

Because some axons and dendrites leave the central nervous system and extend to the surface of the body, flow of fluid within neuron projections may aid the movement of substances from the body's surface to the central nervous system. Examples include the virus of rabies, pseudorabies (a herpesvirus), and agents such as tetanus toxin or the toxins involved in tick paralysis.

Neuroglia

Neurons are greatly outnumbered in the central nervous system by cells of several other types, collectively called **neuroglia** (''nerve glue''). These cells support and give shape to the CNS. Unlike neurons, they can divide and are the source of most tumors of the brain.

A segmented layer of insulation surrounds most axons and some dendrites. The insulating substance is called **myelin**. Myelin is produced by **Schwann cells** for neurons *outside* the CNS and **oligodendrocytes** *in* the CNS. These insulating layers speed impulse conduction, which is discussed below.

Glial cells of the brain place a type of coating around blood **capillaries** (the smallest of blood vessels). This coating creates a separation between the blood and brain, the **blood-brain barrier**, that is not characteristic of other tissues. *The CNS does not exchange substances with blood* in the same way other tissues do. Therefore, it is rather difficult for immune cells to enter the brain area.

NERVE IMPULSES

Cells that are **excitable** (nerve and muscle) must be able to respond to a stimulus and to transmit that response to another site. This depends on properties

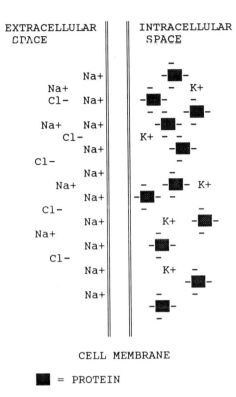

EXTRACELLULAR SPACE

INTRACELLULAR SPACE

CELL MEMBRANE

■ = PROTEIN

Ion Distribution at Cell Membranes A balance of solute particles (osmotic equilibrium) occurs across cell membranes. Because proteins are too large to cross the membrane, but carry many negative charges, an electrical imbalance of charged ions occurs. A membrane potential results from this excess of negative charge on the inside of the membrane.

of the cell membrane and its electric charge. The **electrolytes**, including **sodium**, **potassium**, and **chloride**, and the electrically charged proteins within cells are distributed across the cell's membrane in such a way as to produce the **membrane potential**. This is an electrical force of about 70 mv (millivolts). The outside of the cell membrane is positive relative to the inside of a cell. Sodium (Na^+), potassium (K^+), and chloride (Cl^-) are all managed by **ion pumps** in the cell membrane. These **ions** may also move across a neuron's membrane at sites (**channels**) controlled by **ion gates**.

When an appropriate stimulus (e.g., an electric shock) is applied to a neuron or muscle cell membrane, the ion gates open for a fraction of a second so that Na^+ (abundant on the outside) and K^+ (abundant on the inside) can pulse across the membrane. This collapses the electrical potential momentarily; it is said that the membrane is **depolarized**. This disturbance will depolarize the adjacent membrane area causing a wave of depolarization, much as a length of material will propagate a flame as one area ignites the next. An electrical measurement of depolarization and the immediately following repolarization (as the ion gates are closed and the ion pumps restore the resting potential) will show the **action potential** (also referred to as a nerve **impulse** or the **excitation wave**).

The description of the action potential just given assumes that the nerve membrane was without the myelin sheath. When present, the myelin sheath is regularly interrupted, exposing unmyelinated segments of axon referred to as

nodes of Ranvier. The bare nodes of Ranvier are the only areas where depolarization can occur. When one node undergoes depolarization, electrons flow from one node to the next node, causing the ion gates in the next node to open. In this manner, depolarization moves rapidly along the axon by **saltatory** (jumping) conduction—as fast as 100 meters per second (225 miles per hour).

COMMUNICATION MECHANISMS OF NEURONS

Receptors for Sensations and Stimuli

Four types of specialized receptors receive impulses outside of the CNS. They are classified as **nociceptors**, receptors for pain and aversive stimuli, **chemoreceptors**, **mechanoreceptors**, and **photoreceptors**. Each type of receptor is more sensitive to one type of stimulus than to others.

Each receptor is able to convert the stimulus into an action potential and to rapidly regenerate a **receptor potential**. Thus, if the stimulus is strong, a high frequency of impulses is generated—frequency of impulses is proportionate to the strength of the stimulus.

Receptors may be simple nerve endings or adaptations of nerve endings that are stimulated by heat, cold, touch, etc. Elaborate receptor systems also exist to receive sound (ear), odors (nose structures), visual images (eyes), and taste (taste buds of the tongue). Receptors will be discussed more comprehensively in the chapter Awareness of the Environment and the Special Senses.

Nerve-to-Nerve Connections (Synapses)

Rarely does a single neuron carry an original impulse to its final destination. A chain of many neurons is involved. There is considerable advantage in this arrangement because it allows many connections between neurons. The connections have been shown to be changeable, and this may be a factor in some forms of learning and memory.

The kind of connection between one neuron and another limits the movement of an impulse to only one direction. The connection between neurons is called a **synapse** and is located where an axon terminal knob of one neuron nearly touches the neuron cell body or dendrite of another.

Chemical Communication (Neurotransmitters and Neuromodulators)

It was once assumed that the impulse "jumped" the small synaptic space as a spark might jump from one electric wire to another. However, it is now known that arrival of an impulse causes the release of a biochemical agent, a **neurotransmitter**. The neurotransmitter binds to receptors on the membrane of the next neuron's dendrites or cell body, bringing about change in that mem-

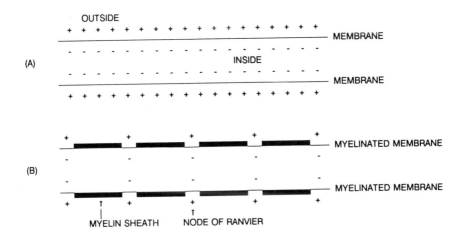

OUTSIDE

INSIDE

(A)

MEMBRANE

MEMBRANE

(B)

MYELINATED MEMBRANE

MYELINATED MEMBRANE

MYELIN SHEATH   NODE OF RANVIER

Nerve Myelin Sheath and Impulse Conduction   Nerve fibers may be (A) nonmyelinated or (B) myelinated. In both cases, the cylindrical nerve fiber is polarized, with the outside positive to the inside. If a point on a membrane is stimulated, depolarization will take place. In (A), a depolarization will disturb adjacent areas, causing a wave of depolarization (the impulse) to travel along the fiber. In (B), only the nodes of Ranvier are polarized. When one node is depolarized, electrical current flows from node to node—a much faster type of impulse conduction.

brane. Therefore, impulses proceed only from axon terminals to dendritic areas of another neuron. In other words, they only go one way.

In addition to neurotransmitters, **neuromodulators** also affect neuron function. A particularly interesting group of neuromodulators contains the **endorphins**, one of which, **beta-endorphin**, is especially interesting. Beta-endorphin appears to cause the so-called ''runner's high'' (an elevated mood associated with exercise) in humans by binding to sites in the brain that also bind morphine.

In addition to these morphine binding sites, brain neuron receptors have been found for lysergic acid diethylamide (LSD), mescaline (from a cactus plant), and other mind-altering drugs. Although specific studies of these actions on dogs is limited, it is reasonable to assume that they probably exist in similar form and function.

Nerve Endings at Muscles and Glands

The cell bodies of motor neurons reside primarily in the central nervous system and reach their target cells, the skeletal muscle, by way of long axons. The terminal knobs engage special sites on muscle fiber membranes to create **motor end plates,** which, like many synapses, secrete acetylcholine (ACh) as a neurotransmitter. One source of fatigue, other than lack of oxygen and metabolic energy, is failure at this junction.

The awful effects of ''nerve gas'' and many insecticides, including some

23

flea sprays, are caused by their ability to block cholinesterase (the enzyme that removes ACh), allowing unbridled stimulation to produce lethal convulsions. The poison produced by the bacterium associated with spoiled foods, *botulinum toxin*, inhibits the release of ACh at synapses and motor end plates. Certain snake venoms exert their actions by binding to ACh receptor proteins.

MUSCLE FIBERS AND MUSCLE CONTRACTION

The electrical properties of muscle have been discussed in this chapter because nervous tissue resembles muscle in this respect. However, the anatomy of muscles, the mechanics of contraction, and other features of muscle are discussed in the chapter The Skeleton and Skeletal Muscles.

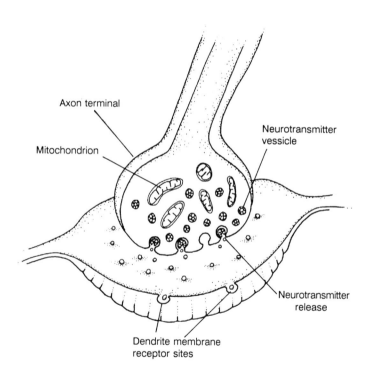

Impulse Condition at Nerve Synapses A synapse consists of an axon terminal in close proximity to a cell body or dendritic membrane of another neuron. The synaptic cleft between them is much narrower than diagrammed; it has the dimension of chemical molecules. The receptor sites on postsynaptic surfaces are specific only for transmitter substances that are released from adjacent axonal endings.

AGING AND DISEASES OF NEURONS AND SYNAPSES—RELATED DYSFUNCTIONS AND DISEASES—AUTOIMMUNE PROBLEMS

As neurons age, they accumulate the pigment **lipofuscin**. Although it was once believed that this resulted in disturbance of neuron function, adequate study has not shown this to be the case.

In fact, it is difficult to claim that individual neurons actually age in some way. However, there is a reduction in their number, especially in certain parts of the brain, and their interconnections are altered. These changes alter memory and the efficiency and speed of learning.

Other changes in neuron function result from reduction in blood supply (perhaps caused by the pressure of nearby tumors), the effects of malnutrition, or the effects of medications, all factors closely allied with aging.

As animals grow older, there is a greater tendency for the **immune** system to malfunction; that is, the immune system fails to recognize some tissue components as belonging to "self." Attacks by the malfunctioning immune system damage the target tissue (see the chapter The Protective Role of the Immune System). Two conditions occur in dogs, humans, and probably some other animals; both also occur in young and old animals.

Multiple sclerosis is an autoimmune condition in which the myelin sheaths of axons and dendrites are injured. A virus of some sort may initiate the process.

Another condition is **myasthenia gravis**. The name suggests grave muscular weakness, but the weakness is secondary. Recent research has shown that an autoimmune attack has occurred against the receptor sites for acetylcholine at neuromuscular connections. This prevents muscle fibrils from being stimulated when an impulse arrives and the neurotransmitter acetylcholine is released. Many times the symptoms of myasthenia are noted in the motor control of the eye and various muscle groups. The symptoms may be varied; faulty control of eye movements, changes in gait, etc., may easily resemble symptoms of other conditions.

A similar situation occurs when a dog is poisoned with certain insecticides, especially those known as **organophosphates**. These chemicals are used because they kill insects by destroying or blocking cholinesterase. Recall that this is the enzyme that removes acetylcholine at synapses so that rapid, repeated impulse transmission can take place normally. If cholinesterase is blocked, the proper functions at synapses cannot occur.

Because electrolyte ions, in proper amounts, are required for maintaining a healthy membrane potential, abnormal electrolyte balances can disrupt the function of excitable tissues. For example, an aging dog being treated with a diuretic, because of a need for the kidneys to excrete more sodium and water, may incidentally excrete inappropriate amounts of potassium. This will result in muscular weakness and ineffective nerve function.

As aging develops, the risk of deterioration of the disks that separate the vertebrae increases, especially in some breeds (e.g., Dachshunds, Beagles, Pekingese). The pressure on nerves leading from the spinal cord produces injury to nerve fibers (see the chapters The Central Nervous System and The Skeleton and Skeletal Muscles).

Hormone imbalances (endocrine disorders) can result in altered neuron function (see the chapter The Endocrine System). A condition called **hyper-adrenocortical myopathy** is characterized by excessive production of steroid hormone from the **adrenal cortex**; this leads to muscle weakness (**myopathy**). Sometimes these steroid hormones are used in older dogs as treatment for in-flammation (e.g., arthritis), and extended use may result in symptoms of this condition. Insufficient **thyroid gland** hormone may be associated with a myop-athy, and, although marked limb dysfunction may not be present, the dog will be intolerant of exercise. However, facial nerve paralysis and carrying the head in a characteristic tilt may be symptomatic. A serious accompanying problem is reduction of motility in the esophagus, resulting in swallowing difficulties. Un-fortunately, treatment with thyroid hormones may be disappointing.

Aging animals have an increased likelihood of developing diabetes. An accompanying symptom may be a reduced function of neuronal tissue (**neurop-athy**). It has been suggested that this condition is related to some alteration in Schwann cells, the cells that provide myelin sheaths to neuron projections. Insulin treatment is used with some success.

4

The Central Nervous System, a Control Center

ORGANIZATION AND FUNCTION

Evolution of the **central nervous system** (CNS) appears to have been a process of adding functionally advanced parts onto preexisting structures. In dogs, some primitive functions have been retained; new levels of sophistication and function have been added. Where new control features were added, they often are characterized by their ability to selectively limit more primitive functions.

Some estimates place the number of neurons in the central nervous system in the trillions; more conservative estimates suggest many billions. Some neurons have thousands of dendritic branches and a great number of axon terminals, creating an enormous range of possible interconnections. Although divided into anatomical areas for discussion (see Table 4.1), all parts of the CNS are intimately connected.

The nervous system serves three categories of function. **Motor activity** refers to muscle activity, gland secretion, etc. **Sensory functions** are conscious or unconscious transfers of information to the CNS. **Association functions** relate to the interchanges of nerve activity between areas of the brain.

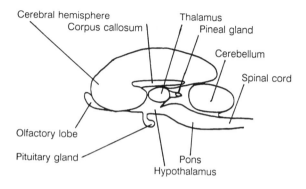

Cerebral hemisphere
Corpus callosum
Thalamus
Pineal gland
Cerebellum
Spinal cord
Olfactory lobe
Pituitary gland
Pons
Hypothalamus

The Dog Brain This diagram illustrates the location of primary parts of the brain. The prespective is of the brain cut straight down its middle, with the view of the inner surface of the right side. An outer surface view would appear different, and it would not allow illustration of several structures that are in the center of the brain.

THE FOREBRAIN

The **forebrain** consists of two general areas. One is called the **telencephalon**. This is made up of the two **cerebral hemispheres** and the **corpus striatum**. The other general area is the **diencephalon**. Its important parts are the **thalamus, hypothalamus**, and **pineal gland**.

Of the above, the cerebral hemispheres are the most advanced portion of the nervous system. This is the major area for information storage (memory), thought and judgment processes, integration of sensory input, and voluntary motor output.

A conspicuous cerebral fiber tract, the **corpus callosum**, is a bridge between the two cerebral hemispheres. Animal and human studies in which the corpus callosum has been cut show that each hemisphere has some unique functions. The right or left brain may show different areas of dominance by one over the other.

Neuronal cell bodies located in the **primary motor area** of the cerebral cortex have direct association with skeletal muscles. However, voluntary muscle action is initiated by other brain areas which stimulate primary motor area neurons. These motor neurons receive projections from adjacent regions of the cortex (especially sensory areas, including visual and auditory areas), from the opposite cerebral hemisphere by way of the corpus callosum, and from lower brain areas, especially the thalamus.

Each **temporal lobe** (on the side of each cerebral cortex) has cortical cells in one group (**auditory sensory area**) that receive auditory signals (from sounds). They are surrounded by an area (**auditory association area**) that distributes these signals for interpretation by other brain areas. Visual discrimination and association are served by the **visual cortex** and its association areas in

TABLE 4.1   Organization of the Central Nervous System

Forebrain
  Telencephalon
  - cerebral hemispheres
  - corpus striatum
  Diencephalon
  - thalamus
  - hypothalamus
  - pineal gland

Brain Stem
  Mesencephalon (midbrain)
  - corpora quadrigemina
  - red nucleus
  - substantia nigra
  - cerebral peduncles
  Rhombencephalon (hindbrain)
  - cerebellum
  - pons
  - medulla oblongata

Spinal Cord
  - cervical
  - thoracic
  - lumbar
  - sacral
  - coccygeal

the **occipital lobes** at the rear of each cerebrum. At the front of each cerebral cortex is the **frontal lobe**. It is composed of groups of neurons that serve the interesting processes of thinking, judging, remembering, and initiating or inhibiting voluntary activity. Loss of these areas or injury to them reveals much of what each does by the alterations in functions that occur. It is not surprising that this area of the brain is exceptionally well developed in humans when compared with dogs.

In dogs and many other animals, the olfactory area is well developed to serve an acute sense of smell. Evidence is accumulating that there also exists here the ability to perceive substances given off by other animals, called **pheromones**, that invoke behavioral responses in a recipient, e.g., mating behavior, aggression, and various hormonelike effects.

The diencephalon, a sort of in-between portion of the brain, is associated with the forebrain and contains three extremely important neuronal structures: the thalamus, the hypothalamus, and the pineal gland.

The thalamus is associated with the cerebral cortex as the entryway for most sensory input except olfaction (smell). The thalamus relays sensory, visual, taste, and tactile signals to higher brain structures. One thalamic pathway is associated with transmission of intense pain. It is probable that thalamic activity is involved in the mental process we call attention, as well as wakefulness and sensory awareness.

The hypothalamus is a truly remarkable, multifunctional structure. It is central to the function of a group of brain areas called the **limbic system**, which includes the thalamus; portions of structures called the **basal ganglia** and parts of the cerebral cortex; the **hippocampus** (a special area of the cerebral cortex); and the nearby **amygdala**, located just below the cortex.

The limbic system is very important to many aspects of behavior and emotions. The limbic system is involved in pleasure sensations, satiety (satisfaction), pain, aversion, and punishment. These responses may be important in the motivation for learning and memory. Variation in the capacity of this system may explain some behavioral differences between otherwise similar dogs. It is significant that the rabies virus is found in the hippocampus and, thus, may disrupt normal behavior.

Tranquilizers, such as chlorpromazine, inhibit the limbic system. Depending on the part of the hypothalamus experimentally stimulated, rage, fear, anxiety, or docility may result.

Other important hypothalamic functions include control of reflexes that maintain body temperature (sweating, shivering, panting), heart rate, blood pressure, hunger and thirst, feeding reflexes, bladder function, and some gastrointestinal activity. The hypothalamus can excite the **reticular activation system**, which controls alertness and wakefulness. Yet some hypothalamic areas, when stimulated, result in sleep.

Hypothalamic activity, in addition to the above, includes production of hormones; in other words, it functions as an endocrine gland, along with a few other brain areas. This unites **neurophysiology** with **endocrinology** to produce the new and productive field of **neuroendocrinology** (see the chapter The Endocrine System).

Malfunction of the hypothalamus may result in a wide variety of metabolic, **autonomic nervous system**, and endocrine effects that strikingly resemble age-related changes. These include alterations in immune function, distribution of body fat, muscle mass, kidney function, glucose metabolism, reproductive status, hormone production, appetite, blood pressure, etc. Some gerontologists wonder if the hypothalamus might deteriorate or become "exhausted" in such a way that its regulatory activities do not function efficiently, accounting for aging. Others believe that the hypothalamus may become variously insensitive to the feedback mechanisms meant for its own control. One theory of aging is actually based on the possible, but not proven, production of a "death hormone" by this gland.

Two complexes of neurons, the amygdala and the hippocampus, are part of the limbic system, as mentioned above. The amygdala is concerned with olfaction (the sense of smell). The hippocampus is especially interesting in regard to aging. Much of its function has come to light because of its implication in **Alzheimer's disease** and memory and learning deficits in humans. Limited study has shown its association with certain sexual phenomena, rage, body movements, and attention to the immediate environment. Electrical stimulation to this area may initiate one type of epileptic seizure that may have olfactory, visual, auditory, and tactile components, at least in humans.

The pineal (pinecone-shaped) gland is located at the back of the midbrain and above the **cerebellum**. It has connections with the CNS that are lost after birth, except for **sympathetic nervous system** connections. In mammals, melatonin has a gonad (sex gland) inhibiting effect (inhibits production of sex hormones) and is believed to adjust reproductive activity to seasons of the year in many species. Recent research has shown that the pineal gland is involved in initiating puberty. This is another example of the close relationship of the nervous system and the endocrine glands.

THE BRAIN STEM

The **brain stem** is primarily, but not exclusively, concerned with unconscious activity. Much of it influences or coordinates essential life processes. For example, the brain stem is involved with respiration, cardiovascular function, wakefulness and sleep, gastrointestinal function, and stereotyped body movement. Coordination of *motor activity* is the special domain of the cerebellum. The brain stem includes areas that coordinate *movements of the eyes, head, and body* that are associated with equilibrium and antigravity support. Some of the brain stem's functions are explained below when its participation in control of the autonomic nervous system is discussed.

The brain stem is composed of the **midbrain** (*mesencephalon*) and **hindbrain** (*rhombencephalon*). Neurons in the mesencephalon coordinate several parts of the brain in controlling wakefulness and sleep. The overall level of CNS activity and the ability to direct attention to conscious functions are related to mesencephalic activity.

The cerebellum is part of the hindbrain and has been called the "silent area" of the brain. If stimulated, no sensations are perceived and motor activity (movement) rarely results. Damaging it does not cause muscle paralysis, but rather smooth, coordinated execution of precise movement (e.g., jumping, running, etc.) is impaired. Thus, the cerebellum monitors activity and has the ability to correct movements even during their execution, a sort of error control.

The **pons** and **medulla oblongata** are involved in control of the autonomic nervous system, which is discussed as a special system. Respiration and cardiovascular functions are regulated by neurons of the pons.

The medulla oblongata, a primitive part of the brain, controls blood pressure, heart rate, secretion of certain glands, and muscular activity of the gastrointestinal tract and urinary bladder.

SLEEP AND WAKEFULNESS

Wakefulness requires a level of activity of the **reticular activating system** (a diffuse system of neurons in the medulla oblongata, pons, mesencephalon, and parts of the diencephalon). A theory of **active sleep** suggests that certain active brain centers (e.g., regions of the hypothalamus) transmit signals to the reticular activating area and initiate sleep by inhibiting the reticular area. At least three areas of the brain can cause sleep when stimulated and insomnia when injured. A theory of **passive sleep** claims that wakefulness is the active state. The reticular activating center seems not only to influence the cerebral cortex but is influenced by it and by peripheral signals from the body. In this theory, input from these sources is thought to initiate wakefulness, and a lack of input is what permits sleep.

SPINAL CORD AND REFLEXES

The only CNS structure seen in many lower animals is a **spinal cord**; they have no conventional brain. The spinal cord is segmented; nerve fibers come and go at regular intervals. Even in higher animal forms, such as the dog, many simple and complex functions still reside only in the spinal cord.

In the dog, the segments are represented by **cervical** (neck) nerves, **thoracic** (chest) nerves, **lumbar** (lower back) nerves, and **sacral** (tail bone) spinal nerves. The total of spinal nerves in dogs is thirty-six to thirty-seven pairs. A number of additional nerve pathways leave the brain without traveling along the spinal cord—the **cranial** nerves to the face, mouth, eyes, vocal cords, etc.

Neurons that originate at sensory receptors and carry action potentials (nerve impulses) toward the CNS are called **afferent** neurons. **Efferent** neurons are those that leave the CNS to interact with peripheral target sites. It is apparent

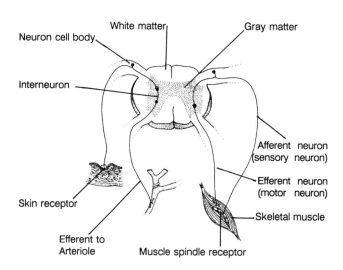

Spinal Reflexes Some important reflexes involve only the spinal cord, but may be influenced by the central nervous system. Afferent and efferent impulses may also communicate within the central nervous system.

that afferent neurons have sensory function and efferent neurons have motor function.

A **spinal reflex arc** is composed of a number of elements. It begins with a sensory receptor and is followed, in order, by an afferent (sensory) neuron that may **synapse** with an efferent (motor) neuron in the spinal cord, and finally, the neuronal junction at the target cell (muscle, gland, etc.). It is common, however, to have one or more **interneurons** between the sensory and motor neurons. This arrangement provides a mechanism for additional connections that distribute impulses to other parts of the spinal cord and brain. Thus, interneurons allow control of a reflex by other areas of the nervous system. Without such inhibition it would not be possible to housebreak a dog so that it learns to wait when the urge to urinate or defecate occurs.

Some reflexes, while executed at the spinal level, have connections by way of ascending spinal tracts to the sensory centers of the cortex that lead to awareness. However, at an involuntary level, there are many spinal reflexes called **visceral reflexes**. Most of these control structures such as blood vessels, bladders, the uterus, intestines, etc. The autonomic nervous system, discussed below, is related to these involuntary reflexes.

THE AUTONOMIC NERVOUS SYSTEM—ANS

This is a special, and generally involuntary, portion of the nervous system. **Autonomic motor nerves** of the autonomic nervous system (ANS) innervate smooth muscle, cardiac (heart) muscle, and glands—all are tissues that are **autonomous**. These tissues are influenced by stimulation but do not need it for function. Their functions may be increased or decreased by nervous activity.

The ANS has two divisions, the **sympathetic** and the **parasympathetic**. Usually, both divisions supply the same tissue but evoke opposite effects. For example, heart rate is increased by sympathetic nerves and decreased by parasympathetic activity.

Acetylcholine (ACh) is the neurotransmitter at synapses connecting one neuron to another in both ANS divisions (see the chapter The Excitable Tissues). Parasympathetic nerve fibers also secrete this transmitter at their endings at target sites of smooth muscle, heart muscle, and glands. However, the sympathetic nerves secrete **norepinephrine** (related to *adrenaline*) at their terminals on glands, smooth muscle, and cardiac muscle. Many drugs and insecticides affect the ANS, as well as the CNS, by altering the function of acetylcholine at synapses. Drugs have been designed to specifically block transmission sites in the ANS.

Sympathetic nerve fibers reach the cells of the central mass of the adrenal gland (**adrenal medulla**). These cells secrete the hormones **epinephrine** and **norepinephrine**, as do the endings of sympathetic neurons. Thus, these hormones act on target tissues in much the same way as sympathetic nerves do. However, these blood-borne hormones have a more prolonged influence on cells with receptors for them.

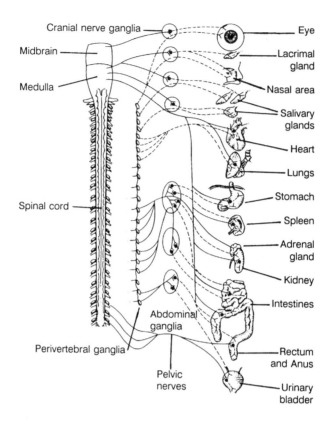

Cranial nerve ganglia — Eye

Midbrain — Lacrimal gland

Medulla — Nasal area

Salivary glands

Heart

Lungs

Spinal cord — Stomach

Spleen

Adrenal gland

Kidney

Intestines

Abdominal ganglia

Perivertebral ganglia — Rectum and Anus

Pelvic nerves — Urinary bladder

The Autonomic Nervous System   The autonomic nervous system (ANS) serves primitive but vital functions. The two divisions, sympathetic (————) and parasympathetic (------), supply nerve fibers to viscera, glands, and a few other tissues. They generally work opposite to one another—one stimulates and the other inhibits the target organ, providing for regulated levels of activity.

CEREBRAL BLOOD FLOW

The brain of an adult dog receives a rather large percentage of the blood in circulation, despite the brain's small percentage of total body weight. Normally, cerebral blood flow is precisely regulated by local reflexes, even though blood pressure may vary. The brain's metabolism is dependent upon high levels of both oxygen and glucose (blood sugar). It is irreparably damaged by loss of either, even for a few minutes. A **stroke** (due to rupture of a blood vessel or a blood clot within a vessel) is one type of brain injury caused by inadequate blood supply. Blows to the head and tumors located in the brain also may affect regional blood flow. Decreased blood flow to the brain results from seriously low blood pressure (as following great blood loss or heart disease), increased intracranial (within the skull) pressure, or blockage of blood vessels to the head. Factors likely to bringabout an increased blood flow to the brain in otherwise healthy dogs include a rise in blood carbon dioxide (CO_2) or a reduction in oxygen (O_2) levels.

THE MENINGES AND CEREBROSPINAL FLUID

Three protective membranes surround the brain and spinal cord. The outer one, attached to the skull and vertebral column, is called the **dura mater** ("hard mother"). The middle layer is called the **arachnoid** ("spider"), containing an extensive network of blood vessels and special cells (the **choroid plexuses**) that secrete the **cerebrospinal fluid**. An inner layer, the **pia mater** ("gentle mother"), directly covers the surface of the brain and spinal cord. These membranes, collectively, are known as the **meninges**, and the fluid between them serves as a shock absorber for the CNS tissue. An infection of these membranes is known as **meningitis**.

The brain has several centrally located cavities(**cerebral ventricles**) which are continuous with the central canal of the spinal cord. **Cerebrospinal fluid** (CSF) is secreted into the cavities, from which it flows to the surface of the brain between the meninges. Sometimes samples of CSF are removed for diagnosis of disease.

Certain **neuroglial** cells (**astrocytes**) surround blood capillaries in the brain with an extra membrane (see the chapter The Excitable Tissues). This separates the blood from the brain's tissue to a greater degree than from other tissue fluid spaces. The CSF is not a filtrate of the blood (its components are actually secreted by cells located in the richly vascularized choroid plexuses), thus the CSF has a different composition than the blood plasma, and many substances cannot enter the CSF.

This has given rise to the concept of the **blood-brain barrier**, a generally useful situation since it *protects* the brain from many toxic substances. The blood-brain barrier does not restrict glucose, alcohols, and steroid hormones, but many *other substances are denied* entrance, such as many normal metabolic products and a number of drugs (e.g., the antibiotics **gentamicin** and **neomycin**). Drugs needed for treatment of the brain must be appropriately selected by the veterinarian in order to effectively reach the CSF.

AGE AND THE NERVOUS SYSTEM

Since the nervous system has a central role in perceiving the environment through sight, smell, hearing, and taste, and responding to it through movement, cognition, and communication, it becomes obvious when age reduces its efficiency. Reduced sensory awareness acutely affects the quality of any animal's life.

Aging and Brain Size

A reduction in brain size accompanies aging. Both gray and white matter are lost, and with great age, cerebral cortical cell loss occurs. However, some brain areas show little or no loss at all. Recent animal research suggests that some of the loss in brain mass may be a result of low levels of brain usage; increasing the amount of stimulus from the environment was able to prevent much of such loss in rats.

Aging Neurons and Synapses

Neural cell branches (**dendritic arbor**) in the cerebral cortex markedly diminish with age. There is also a reduction in the neurotransmitters that are required by neuron connections. However, some dendrites may develop more branches and rearrange their connections. This **neuronal plasticity** may offset some of the effects of neuron loss.

When nerve trunks are cut, but their neuron cell bodies remain intact, regrowth of some branches (axons and dendrites) restores some peripheral nerve function, and synaptic remodeling occurs in the central nervous system.

As animals age, remodeling may occur at a slower rate. As loss of neurons accompanies aging, the loss is offset to the degree that some kind of repair, including this remodeling, takes place.

One significant study compared the rate at which various brain tissues of Beagles were able to use blood sugar (glucose). The frontal area of the cerebral cortex showed a progressive decline from that seen at three years of age to almost half that value at ages fourteen to sixteen years. Other areas also showed lower glucose utilization with age, while some showed no meaningful change.

Lipofuscin is a darkly pigmented deposit increasingly found in aging cells, including neurons. Below normal oxygen levels (**hypoxia**) and vitamin E deficiency correspond with production of this pigment, but no convincing evidence supports the view that this age-related pigment destroys cells or their function.

Sleep Disorders

The amount and pattern of sleep varies with a dog's age. Elderly dogs may have sleep difficulties as a consequence of many neurological, endocrine, and metabolic disorders. Possible factors in sleep disorders are **hypoglycemia** (low blood sugar), **hypothyroidism** (low thyroid activity), uremia (high blood levels of urea, sometimes caused by kidney dysfunction), liver malfunction, and **hypercapnia** (high blood carbon dioxide).

Sleep apnea (halts in breathing during sleep) may result in inadequate sleep. Loud snoring is common in some older dogs. It may accompany sleep apnea, demonstrating the role that respiratory obstruction may play in the condition. Drugs may complicate this condition and cardiovascular complications may result from it.

Periodic movements in sleep (**myoclonus**) are associated with aging. Uncontrolled jerking and other movements may be observed in patterns that exceed the more familiar movements seen in younger animals during sleep.

NERVOUS SYSTEM DISEASES

Central Nervous System (CNS) Neuron Loss and Function

Because dogs do not have the same verbal activity as humans or the same level of thought process, many CNS diseases in humans are not described in the veterinary literature. However, older dogs and rats are the only nonprimates known to have lesions (**neuritic plaques**) in their brains that resemble those seen in **Alzheimer's** disease. Further research may shed more light on the significance of this finding.

However, loss of neurons and reflex function does occur in all aging mammals. This places all of them at greater risk of accidents, from the failure to see or hear an oncoming car to being unable to defend against attacks.

Depression

The term *depression* is sometimes used when referring to dog behavior. It relates to a dog's unresponsiveness to being called or to invitations to play, eat, etc. Research has not provided clear knowledge that a parallel exists between this and depression in humans. In any case, older dogs do show less responsiveness generally, and changes in the CNS may be reasonable causes.

Demyelinization

Loss of the nerve fiber's myelin sheath occurs with some diseases of aging animals. This slows impulse conduction to a serious degree. In humans with Alzheimer's disease there is a decrease in myelin in certain brain regions, not in others. In some conditions, **demyelinization** results from an autoimmune attack on the myelin sheaths, further discussed in the chapter The Protective Role of the Immune System.

Stroke

Loss of blood flow to a specific area of the brain is called a *stroke*. It can be caused by a ruptured blood vessel or blockage of the vessel by a blood clot. Fortunately, stroke, which increases with age, is less common in dogs than in humans. Stroke may not be a single process. Blockages or hemorrhages may occur at different times, accumulating over time. The occurrence of stroke increases with age.

Degenerative Myelopathy

The age-related condition **degenerative myelopathy** is associated with degeneration of white matter (nerve fiber tracts) in the thoracic region of the spinal cord. Hind limb weakness, unsteadiness (ataxia), and turning under of the hind feet are symptoms of this poorly understood condition. It is common in German Shepherds, but other breeds are susceptible. The primary cause and an effective treatment are unknown.

Vertebral Injury and Degeneration

Intervertebral disk disease, fibrocartilaginous emboli, spondylosis deformans, and **dural ossification** are the veterinary terms that describe altered conditions in the vertebral bone or disks. Degeneration results in secondary injury to the spinal cord or nerves as they emerge through the spaces between the vertebrae. Paralysis and loss of sensation commonly occur in the body areas affected. Pain may be a major concern, along with the loss of locomotion and control of the urinary bladder and bowel. Long-bodied dogs seem more susceptible, but the conditions are not exclusive to them. When treated early, good results are often produced.

Horner's Syndrome

Horner's syndrome is a set of symptoms that follow some injuries to the autonomic nervous system. The eye shows prominent symptoms: the eyelid droops, the **nictitating membrane** or third eyelid protrudes, and the pupil of the affected eye is constricted. Causes vary, but they include injury to the upper spinal cord at areas that contain ANS fibers. Sometimes a middle ear infection is associated with the condition. This condition is not age-specific, but older dogs may be more prone to accidental injuries.

Secondary Brain Malfunction

Substances that affect nervous system function may occur as a result of the failure of other organ systems. As dogs age, their livers and kidneys do not function as well. Toxins that the liver would have ordinarily dealt with or substances that would have been excreted by a healthy kidney may now accumulate. Metabolic disorders, such as those accompanying **diabetes mellitus** (e.g., high blood levels of **ketones**), may also cause nervous tissue to function less adequately. Veterinary attention is likely to include dietary controls as well as medications for the primary organ failure.

Brain Disease Caused by Treatment of Other Conditions

Treatment-caused disease conditions are said to be **iatrogenic** and are probably quite common in older dogs that are under treatment for some medical condition. The side effects of many drugs may lead to a wide array of symptoms that are preventable and treatable. **Hypoglycemia** (low blood sugar), **hypothyroidism** (low thyroid hormone), or impaired delivery of oxygen to the brain may cause or contribute to states of confusion sometimes seen in older dogs.

5

Awareness of the Environment and the Special Senses

THE **SPECIAL SENSES** are vision, hearing (**audition**), taste (**gustation**), and smell (**olfaction**). These are all well developed in dogs, with the sense of smell being notable as compared with humans. Receptors for these senses have unique features among nervous system tissues. They are relatively specific. A given type of receptor has a much greater response to one type of stimulus as compared with others.

The olfactory receptors in the nose respond to minute amounts of airborne chemicals, substances that are unlikely to stimulate other receptors even if they had access to them. Receptors in the retina of the eye respond to extremely small amounts of light.

Each of the four special senses is represented in the brain by separate areas. For example, the retina's neuron fibers go to the visual cortex at the rear of the brain. This arrangement allows recognition of the pattern of stimuli, e.g., bits of light from the field of view. When a stimulus is applied, receptors respond with bursts of impulses that are proportional to the strength of the stimulus. That is how quantitative information is generated.

STRUCTURE AND FUNCTION

THE EYE AND VISUAL CORTEX

The eye is somewhat round, with three layers of tissue. The outer layer is tough, fibrous connective tissue modified at the clear front portion, the **cornea**. The inner layer, the **retina**, is composed of nerve tissue and photoreceptors. The middle layer, the **choroid**, contains many blood vessels and is located behind the retina. The retina receptors are connected by the optic nerve to the visual cortex of the brain. The **posterior chamber** of the eye is filled with a jellylike **vitreous humor**. A smaller **anterior chamber**, in front of the lens, contains clear fluid, the **aqueous humor**.

The cornea is the first surface where **refraction** (bending) of light rays occurs. At the rear of the anterior chamber, **ligaments** (suspending fibers) hold the lens in place. The choroid, or vascular layer, continues in the front of the eye as a pigmented **iris**. Its pigment determines the eye color and the round opening in the iris is the **pupil** of the eye.

The lens is clear, curved outward on both sides, and somewhat elastic. Its attachment ligaments are associated with small muscles that are able to flatten the lens. Light beams are focused on the retina by first being refracted at the cornea and then by the adjustable curve of the lens.

Photoreceptor cells in the retina called **rods** contain chemical molecules that are easily altered by light. Light energy causes a series of chemical changes in the receptors. These changes release energy that sends bursts of impulses according to the amount of light. Rod function is enhanced by a membrane that lies behind the rods called the **tapetum lucidum**. This membrane causes the eyes of dogs and many other animals to "shine" back at a light—and appear red in photographs. Dogs also have the ability to see movement quite easily, although they seem unable to see fixed objects very well.

A second type of receptor called a **cone** has a different photopigment that provides sensitivity to colors. Bright light is required for these receptors. Dogs have few cones and are considered relatively color-blind.

Visual signals reach the brain by way of **optic nerves**. Visual problems can arise in several parts of the eye, injury to the optic nerve pathway, or failure of the parts of the brain (visual cortex) that receive and process visual information.

Movements of an eye are controlled by sets of muscles that are arranged to pull the eye in any direction. In humans, they are coordinated so that both eyes have substantially overlapped fields of view. Dogs have less overlap in their fields of view because their eyes are not positioned as far forward in the head. The flat-faced breeds' eyes (e.g., Bulldogs) are more forward. Visual overlap is needed for **binocular** (two-eyed or three-dimensional) vision to measure distance and shape.

The positioning of the eyes to the side of the head does provide a much wider field of view to the sides. The movement of the eyes is controlled by voluntary and involuntary reflexes, including signals from the balance elements of the inner ear.

THE EAR AND AUDITORY FUNCTION

The most familiar function of the ear is auditory. This sense is very well developed in the dog. Dogs are able to hear sounds of higher frequency (e.g., other animal sounds and silent dog whistles), and sounds too soft to be heard easily by humans (e.g., the familiar sound of the family car nearing its home).

Vibrations of air molecules against the eardrum (**tympanic membrane**), are amplified by small middle ear bones (**ossicles**), which then stimulate receptor cells in the **cochlea** of the inner ear. Cells in different areas of the cochlea are stimulated by different vibration frequencies.

It has been claimed that hearing loss in old dogs frequently precedes a loss of vision. However, in a stable environment the inability to hear is not so readily noticed until sight is lost.

The inner ear also contains the **vestibular apparatus**, which allows a dog to sense body position relative to the direction of gravity and movement. Fluid in **semicircular canals** moves in response to body movement and stimulates special hair cells. The projecting hairs, affected by the fluid movement, transmit this to their receptor cells.

THE SENSE OF SMELL

The sense of smell (olfaction) is mediated by receptors in the nose. The dog's ability to smell and to recognize very faint odors is highly developed, perhaps a million times greater than in humans. In fact, a great deal of communication between dogs is done with this sense. The recognition of a bitch in heat is one example. Dogs experience a medley of odors in a bowl of food that appears quite unimpressive to humans. The part of the dog's brain dedicated to processing olfactory information is many times larger than in humans.

Olfaction relies on several receptors, each having a different sensitivity to about seven classes of substances. Whenever airborne molecules dissolve in the moist membranes within the nose, receptors are stimulated. Because the number of odors that can be distinguished, at least in man, may be in the hundreds, the brain must have a mechanism that blends combinations of these stimuli into an "odor image."

An interesting area of research shows that dogs and many other animals release substances into the air, to which another animal of the same species may respond, but these substances are not actually odors and may not be perceived as a smell. These substances are called **pheromones** and influence interaction between individuals. Pheromones are particularly important in aggressive and sexual behavior.

THE TONGUE AND THE SENSE OF TASTE

Taste buds (taste receptors) for several tastes are distributed on regions of the tongue. In the human, at least, it is known that there are four different types of these receptors that distinguish sweet, salt, sour, and bitter. Of course, it is difficult to design an experiment to test such responses in the dog. As with smell, many categories of taste may be a result of the brain's powers of association as it responds to combinations of taste stimuli.

AGING AND DISEASES OF THE SPECIAL SENSES

THE AGING EYE

The proteins of the lens change with age; lens elasticity is considerably reduced. The more rigid lens cannot be easily flattened, and will not so readily assume a greater curvature. This loss of flexibility is called **presbyopia**.

The pupil of the aging eye is less able to dilate or constrict to adjust the amount of light admitted. Normally, brighter light reflexively reduces the diameter of the pupil, improving the sharpness of retinal images. On the other hand, reduced light normally results in reflex dilation of the pupil, which allows more light to enter the eye.

Ultraviolet light (e.g., from sunlight) produces yellowing in the lens. Furthermore, other chemical changes in lens composition may produce opacities (cloudiness) and reduce clarity. These changes are called **cataracts**. Cataracts are common in dogs with untreated diabetes. Specifically inherited cataracts also occur. *Some changes in lens proteins occur without other apparent causes and seem to be true age effects.* Cataracts reduce the amount of light that passes through the lens, and light is deflected by the opacities, which interferes with visual contrast between parts of the image.

Another age-related condition results in the eye globe becoming shrunken. This is associated with some cataracts. The reason for the wasting (**atrophy**) of the globe appears to be an autoimmune attack on parts of the eye, the lens, and the tissues of the iris. The eye lens is normally isolated from the individual dog's immune system. Lack of contact causes the immune system to fail to "learn" that the lens proteins are part of "self." If lens proteins are released by injury or disease, an inappropriate immune response may cause damage to the lens.

It is important to note that the lens of the eyes of older dogs undergo a process that causes them to appear hazy. This condition is called **lenticular sclerosis** (*or* **nuclear sclerosis**). *It is a common condition that does not appear to degrade vision. To an observer, the hazy appearance may erroneously be considered cataract formation.*

The aqueous humor fluid of the eye is produced by a part of the **ciliary body**. A canal is present by which it is drained back into the bloodstream—this is not tears. In elderly dogs this drainage may become impaired. If so, inner eye pressure is increased, and **glaucoma** develops. In some cases, **lens luxation**, a dislocation of the lens caused by weakening of the supporting fibers, may block drainage. The pressure, pressing on the blood vessels in the eye, reduces the blood supply to the retina, causing retinal degeneration and blindness. The condition sometimes develops without notable early symptoms. Acute glaucoma, on the other hand, is quite painful, calling for immediate veterinary care.

Degeneration of the central region (**macular region**) of the retina results in a loss of central vision (**central progressive retinal atrophy**—CPRA). This is the part of the retina that accounts for the sharpest vision. It seems to be related to some disease process of the blood vessels in the choroid, with secondary alterations of the retina and pigmented layer. There are no known preventative measures or treatments; the initial cause is unknown.

Overall degeneration of the retina (**progressive retinal atrophy**—PRA) also results in a loss of vision. Many breeds are susceptible. The characteristic loss of night vision causes an affected dog to fear activity in low-lighted areas. Although seen in older dogs, PRA usually has its onset in the middle-aged dog.

Enophthalmia refers to a receding of the eyeball into the eye socket. This condition may result in **entropion**, an inversion of the edge of the eyelid, particularly the lower one. A common complication is ulceration of the cornea because of abrasion as the lid rubs against it.

Some old dogs lose the ability to fully close their eyelids (**lagophthalmos**). This condition is a result of damage to the seventh cranial nerve and may also be associated with facial paralysis. The eye surface (cornea) is damaged by exposure.

The cornea of an older dog is sometimes damaged by abrasion because of lack of adequate tear formation. In other cases, the corneal cells themselves may undergo changes (**dystrophy**) with age that interfere with adequate water content of the corneal cell layers.

A dramatic corneal disease in very old dogs has an equally impressive title: **canine geriatric superficial corneal dystrophy**. It is characterized by deposits of calcium in the cornea. Accompanying this condition is notable tear formation and extreme distress from exposure to bright light (**photophobia**). With time, the cornea becomes opaque and ulcers form on it. Although the reason is unknown, this disease is accompanied by **dementia**.

Many medical disorders are associated with or cause changes in the visual apparatus. **Cushing's disease**, caused by excessive production of hormones from the cortex of the adrenal gland, has widespread effects on body metabolism, blood pressure, etc. Other conditions that may have a connection to eye changes are some cancers, thyroid malfunction, diabetes mellitus, heartworm infestation, and bacterial infections of the eye.

DEAFNESS AND DISEASES OF THE EAR

Older dogs commonly experience a reduced ability to hear (**presbycusis**). Damage to the small bones within the ear (**ossicles**) by calcium deposits or trauma to the tympanic membrane by rupture or injury from infection may result in conduction deafness, a common accompaniment to aging. As deafness progresses, some dogs retain an ability to hear high frequencies as in a loud whistle.

So-called nerve deafness may have various causes. Hearing receptors, if damaged by infection or physical injury, may be at fault. Also, the problem may be failure of the **vestibulocochlear nerve**, which is the route to the auditory centers of the brain, or various pathways in the brain involved with processing auditory information.

The dog's ear, those of drop-eared breeds in particular, is shaped to invite injury and infection. Parasites, such as **ear mites**, find the external ear canal an ideal living site. A number of bacteria, fungi, and yeasts also infect the external ear. The older dog may be more susceptible to these infections; the older dog is certainly less tolerant of such health threats.

Otitis media (infection of the middle ear) can arise when infection of the **eustachian tube**, a connection between the middle ear and the throat compartment, travels to the middle ear. Infection in the outer ear (**otitis externa**) can spread into the middle ear by way of a ruptured eardrum.

If infection or other injury occurs in the internal ear, deafness can result and the dog's sense of balance may be disturbed. In this case, as well as those mentioned above, pain is likely. The dog will shake its head and rotate the head toward the affected side. It may be unwilling to eat and drink, and a defect in gait may include turning in circles.

LOSS OF THE SENSE OF SMELL

Loss of olfaction may accompany aging and reduce the recognition and pleasure of food flavors.

Breathing through the nose may become impaired in older dogs as nasal growths such as **polyps** and **tumors** become evident. The same is true when infections in the nose and sinuses are present. Obviously, such conditions affect the ability to smell.

LOSS OF THE SENSE OF TASTE

The ability to taste may be reduced in aging dogs, as it is in humans, by loss of **taste buds** on the tongue. The degree to which this occurs or the extent that it may affect a dog's life is not defined by any adequate study.

6

The Endocrine System: Hormones and Chemical Control

T HE BODY has two glandular systems. One system (the **exocrine** glands) consists of cells associated with ducts through which secreted products are collected and delivered to other sites. These products do not control the function of other cells. Examples are sweat glands on the foot pads of dogs, salivary glands, and the part of the pancreas that produces digestive enzymes.

The subject of this chapter is the **endocrine system**, sometimes referred to as the **ductless gland system**. Products of these glands (**hormones**) are delivered directly into the bloodstream in order to reach target tissues. Target cells possess mechanisms whereby they recognize a hormone that they would otherwise ignore. The endocrine glands, their target tissues, and their effects are presented in Table 6.1.

THE NATURE AND ORIGIN OF HORMONES

Hormones take many forms. Some are chains of amino acids (**peptides),** slightly modified single amines (**monoamines) or diamines** (two joined amines), and others belong to different chemical classes altogether. The **steroid hormones** are classified with fats. Another group, the **prostaglandins**, consists of modified fatty acids.

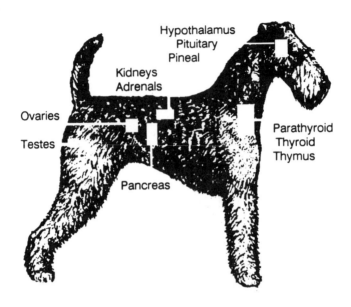

Location of Major Endocrine Glands The major endocrine glands are in the areas indicated. Several glands are quite near one another, e.g., parathyroid, thyroid, and thymus. The typical male glands (testes) and female glands (ovaries) are shown on the one figure. Hormone glands located in the intestinal tract are not illustrated.

The **ovaries**, **testes**, **adrenal cortex**, and the **fetal-placental unit** are sites of steroid hormone production. Many enzymes needed for their synthesis are present in these tissues. Steroids are produced from **cholesterol**, which is readily synthesized for that purpose by the body. All steroid hormones are similar except for small chemical differences.

Peptide hormones are produced by the **hypothalamus, anterior pituitary gland, parathyroid gland, pancreas, kidney**, and **gastrointestinal tract**. Because of their small size and well-defined structures, many of these hormones can now be produced by laboratory methods. **Insulin** from the pancreas is large enough to be considered a small protein.

The **thyroid gland**, the **pineal gland**, and the **adrenal medulla** produce hormones that are derivatives of amino acids. Thyroid hormone, for example, is a combination of two molecules of **tyrosine** (an amino acid) with three or four **iodine** atoms added.

Virtually all tissues produce **prostaglandins** from specific fatty acids. Since their action is local, they are sometimes referred to as **paracrine secretions** rather than hormones.

The small size of hormones makes them susceptible to loss by urinary excretion. Many hormones, modified or intact, are excreted; their metabolic activity may be estimated by their abundance in the urine and their concentration in the blood.

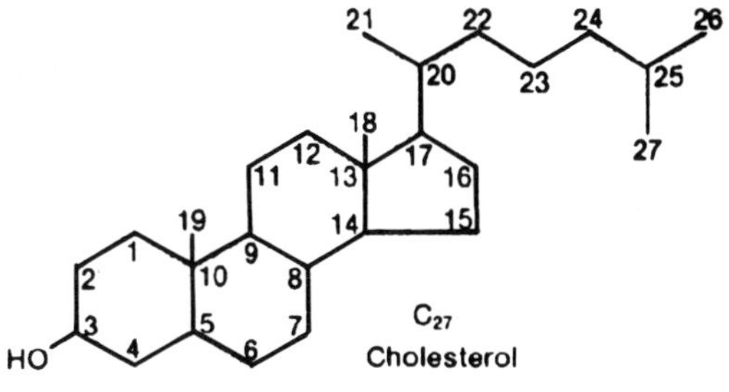

21 **22** **24** **26**
20 **23** **25**
27

18
12
11 **13** **17**
16
19 **9** **8**
1 **10** **14** **15**
2
3 **5** **7**
4 **6**

HO

C_{27}
Cholesterol

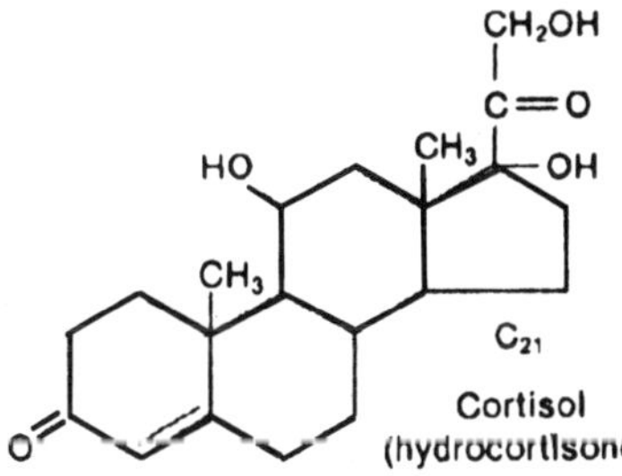

CH_2OH
$C=O$
CH_3 OH
HO

CH_3

O

C_{21}

Cortisol
(hydrocortisone)

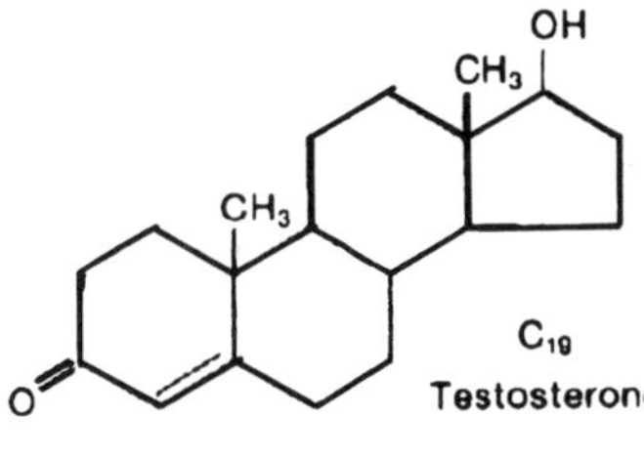

OH
CH_3
CH_3

O

C_{19}
Testosterone

OH
CH_3

HO

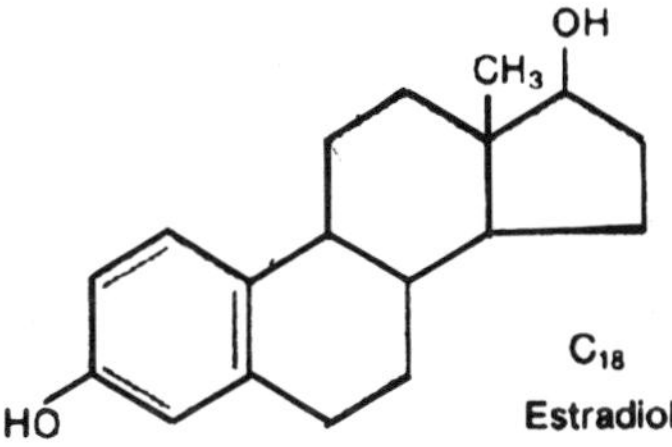

C_{18}
Estradiol

Cholesterol and Steroid Hormones   Cholesterol is the forerunner of all the steroid hormones. Also, slight differences between steroid molecules yield extremely different biological properties. Carbon atoms and hydrogen atoms exist at each numbered junction in the structures shown.

TABLE 6.1 Hormones and Their Effects

Gland	Hormones	Target tissues	General effects
Adrenal cortex	Glucocorticoids (e.g., cortisol)	Many tissues, especially muscles and liver	Glucose and amino acid metabolism
	Mineralocorticoids (e.g., aldosterone)	Kidney tubules	Na^+ reabsorption, K^+ excretion
Adrenal medulla	Epinephrine	Cardiac muscle; smooth muscle of bronchioles and blood vessels; liver	Forceful blood vessel contraction; dilation of bronchioles; raises blood pressure, blood glucose, and blood fatty acids
	Norepinephrine	Similar to epinephrine	Forceful, generalized vasoconstriction; otherwise similar to epinephrine, with weaker effects
Hypothalamus	Releasing and inhibiting hormones (e.g., CRH, GnRH, PIF, TRH, GRH, somatostatin—*see text*)	Anterior pituitary	Regulates production and release of anterior pituitary hormones
	Antidiuretic hormone (ADH)	Kidney tubules, smooth muscles of blood vessels	Enhances water conservation by enabling water reabsorption; vasoconstriction; released at posterior pituitary
	Oxytocin	Smooth muscle of uterus, mammary glands	Uterine contraction; contraction of mammary gland milk ducts
Intestine (small)	Secretin	Pancreas	Stimulates water and bicarbonate secretion; enhances cholecystokinin action on pancreas
	Cholecystokinin (CCK)	Gallbladder and pancreas	Empties gallbladder; production of pancreatic enzymes and pancreatic secretion; maintains pancreatic exocrine cells
	Gastric inhibitory peptide (GIP)	Stomach; islets of Langerhans (pancreas)	Inhibits gastric emptying and secretion; stimulates insulin secretion

TABLE 6.1 Hormones and Their Effects (*continued*)

Gland	Hormones	Target tissues	General effects
Islets of Langer-hans (pancreas)	Insulin	Most tissues	Promotes cellular uptake of glucose and amino acids; glycogen and fat synthesis by cells
	Glucogon	Most tissues	Promotes fat and glycogen break-down (lysis); gener-ally opposite to insulin actions
Ovaries	Estrogen	Uterus; mammary glands	Induces uterine and endometrial growth; causes secondary female sexual char-acteristics to de-velop
	Progesterone	Uterus; mammary glands	Promotes matura-tion of mammary glands for milk pro-duction; brings about uterine changes, especially affecting the muscle during pregnancy
Parathyroid	Parathyroid hor-mone (PTH)	Bone, intestine, and kidneys	Increases Ca^{++} removal (resorption) from bone; en-hances renal Ca^{++} reabsorption; acts to raise blood calcium
Pineal gland	Melatonin	Hypothalamus and an-terior pituitary gland	Affects secretion of gonadotropins; may initiate puberty
Pituitary, anterior	Adrenocorti-cotrophic hormone (ACTH)	Trophic hormone to the adrenal cortex	Stimulates secretion of glucocorticoids
	Follicle stimulating hormone (FSH), a gonadotropin	Trophic hormone to the gonads (overies or tes-tes)	Promotes steroid (estrogen or tes-tosterone) produc-tion; required for production of ova or sperm
	Luteinizing hor-mone (LH), a gonad-otropin	Trophic hormone to the gonads (overies or tes-tes)	Develops corpus luteum and stimu-lates progesterone production by ova-ries; participates in gamete production
	Thyroid stimulating hormone (TSH)	Trophic hormone to the thyroid gland	Causes secretion of thyroid hormones

TABLE 6.1 Hormones and Their Effects (*continued*)

Gland	Hormones	Target tissues	General effects
	Prolactin	Mammary glands	Induces milk formation
	Growth Hormone (GH)	Most tissue	Protein synthesis and growth; lipolysis; increased blood glucose
Pituitary, posterior (see hypothalamus, above)	ADH and oxytocin are produced in the hypothalamus and released by the posterior pituitary		
Stomach	Gastrin	Stomach	Stimulates acid secretion by appropriate stomach cells
Testes	Testosterone	Prostate gland, seminal vesicles, and other organs	Causes development of male secondary sexual characteristics; promotes aggressiveness and sexual drive
Thymus	Thymosins	Lymph nodes	Influences lymphocyte differentiation into specific types
Thyroid gland	Thyroxine (T_4) and triiodothryronine (T_3)	Most tissues	Stimulates growth and development; stimulates cell metabolic rate and O_2 consumption

Hormone molecules that are very *similar* in chemical structure may have very *different* biological functions. A good example is provided by the steroid hormones where a large molecule such as **testosterone** determines the maleness of an individual. However, by the addition of a single hydrogen atom, testosterone becomes the female sex hormone **estradiol**. With slightly greater modification, a testosterone molecule will no longer be a sex steroid at all but will change to **aldosterone**, which acts on kidney cells to moderate their handling of sodium ions.

HOW HORMONES WORK

No cell responds to a hormone unless it has some way to recognize its presence and react to it. One of the best understood mechanisms is called the **second messenger system**. Some cells with specific **binding sites** on their cell membranes bind *specific* hormones. The hormone is considered a **first messenger**. The act of binding to its specific membrane receptor causes the production of a **second messenger** within the cell.

In several instances, the second messenger is a breakdown product of **adenosine triphosphate** (ATP). Binding of the hormone stimulates conversion of ATP into a form of **adenosine monophosphate** (AMP) called **cyclic AMP** (cAMP), the second messenger itself. Cyclic AMP may stimulate a number of cell functions.

Steroid hormones operate via another mechanism. As fats they readily cross the lipoidal (fatty) cell membrane. Membrane receptors are not present for these hormones. However, target cells must have cytoplasmic proteins with binding affinity for specific steroid hormones. Some steroids also localize in small amounts in specific brain areas, providing a mechanism for their influence on neural activity and behavior.

CONTROL OF HORMONE PRODUCTION AND RELEASE

If a hormone directly affects the production of another hormone, it is said to be a **tropic** (or **trophic**) hormone. The anterior pituitary gland produces several such hormones. **Thyrotropin**, for example, causes the thyroid gland to release thyroid hormone. Other hormones from the hypothalamus are tropic to the anterior pituitary and control its function.

Regulation of hormone production and release is provided by **feedback systems**. In some cases, hormones themselves inhibit further production by acting on the gland of their origin. In other cases, hormones inhibit production of tropic hormones upon which their synthesis and release depends. Such feedback loops represent ways that hormone levels or their actions are monitored and the information is used to regulate endocrine gland function.

THE HYPOTHALAMIC-PITUITARY RELATIONSHIP

The **pituitary gland** was considered the "master" gland because of its profound influence on many other glands.

Research has now shown that the pituitary has a master, the **hypothalamus**, a brain structure emphasized in the chapter The Central Nervous System. The hypothalamus produces **releasing hormones** (or **factors**) that stimulate the anterior pituitary. These releasing hormones are: (1) **growth hormone releasing hormone** (GHRH), (2) **adrenocorticotropic releasing hormone** (CRH), (3) **thyrotropin releasing hormone** (TRH), and (4) **gonadotropin releasing hormone** (GnRH).

Certain products of the hypothalamus control by *inhibiting, rather than stimulating*, pituitary hormone production. One of these, **prolactin inhibiting factor** (PIF), inhibits prolactin release. Another hypothalamic product, **somatostatin**, inhibits the secretion of growth hormone by the anterior pituitary gland.

These **neuroendocrine** substances are significant because through them the brain has extensive control of bodily functions. The action of many hormones on the brain also allows mood and behavioral influences. The hypothalamus is also a site where body processes may be modified by mental states such as stress.

EFFECTS OF AGE AND DISEASE ON ENDOCRINE GLANDS AND HORMONES

THE POSTERIOR PITUITARY

The **posterior pituitary** is the rearmost portion of the pituitary gland, and contains two hormones actually produced in the hypothalamus by neurons. Axons transport the hormones and release them to the bloodstream. The two posterior pituitary hormones are **oxytocin** and **antidiuretic hormone** (ADH).

Oxytocin stimulates smooth muscle. For example, it may act on the uterus, enhancing its contractions during the birth process. Oxytocin also promotes contraction of the ducts in the **mammary glands** (breasts), bringing about milk letdown. Most people have observed that kittens and puppies "knead" their mother's breast with their paws while suckling. Kneading stimulates nerve receptors in the nipple area of mammals, sending nerve impulses to the hypothalamus to stimulate the production and release of oxytocin.

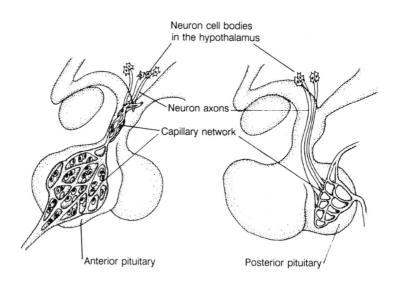

Anatomy of the Pituitary Gland Several releasing hormones (peptide molecules) are produced by hypothalamic neurons and carried, by a special blood capillary system, to the anterior pituitary (a) where they influence the production of several hormones. The hypothalamus also produces two peptide hormones, oxytocin and antidiuretic hormone (ADH). These are carried by neuronal axons to the posterior pituitary where they are released.

Antidiuretic hormone is a powerful **vasoconstrictor** (causing constriction of small blood vessels), hence the name **vasopressin**. Actually, there are several vasopressins. One form, **arginine** vasopressin, acts on cells of the kidney, facilitating the **osmotic** passage of water back into the blood when sodium is conserved by reabsorption.

The body has a system of cells (**osmoreceptors**) that react to the concentration of sodium chloride (NaCl) in the blood. These osmoreceptors cause the release of ADH whenever the blood concentration of NaCl is too high or the blood pressure is too low. By conserving body water via kidney function, the high NaCl concentration is offset, and the blood pressure is better sustained by conserving a normal blood volume.

When ADH is not sufficient, a condition called **diabetes insipidus** occurs. This is characterized by excessive urine volume. Sodium is not properly retained and the water associated with it is lost. The chapter The Urinary System deals with the function of ADH in more detail.

Aged dogs often show dysfunctions in fluid and **electrolyte** balance, and malfunction of the posterior pituitary hormone system may be responsible.

THE ANTERIOR PITUITARY

The forward portion (**anterior pituitary gland**) produces six different hormones and is controlled by the hypothalamic releasing hormones discussed above. Four of these are tropic hormones that exert control over the **gonads** (testes and ovaries), **adrenal cortex**, and **thyroid gland**. The other two are **growth hormone** and **prolactin**.

There are two **gonadotropins: follicle stimulating hormone** (FSH) and **luteinizing hormone** (LH). FSH acts on the ovaries to induce maturing of an **ovarian follicle** that contains an **ovum** (egg). In the male, it influences sperm production. In addition to these cellular effects, FSH causes ovarian production of the female hormone **estrogen** or the testicular production of the male **testosterone**.

Luteinizing hormone (LH) is the agent that causes release of an egg and production of the pregnancy-associated steroid, **progesterone**. In the male, LH is also needed for sperm and testosterone production. Age-related changes in gonadotropins and sex steroids are also discussed in the chapter The Reproductive System.

Thyrotropin (also called **thyroid stimulating hormone**, or TSH) stimulates the thyroid gland. No age-related alterations in blood level of thyrotropin have been observed.

The anterior pituitary glands of mammals, and a small central portion of the pituitary in dogs, also produce **corticotropin** (ACTH). It regulates production of the steroids of the adrenal cortex. The term *cortex* refers to the outer layer of a structure; the *medulla* is the inner portion of a structure.

Older dogs may more frequently have **adenomas** (gland tissue cancer) of the pituitary that secretes excess corticotropin. Boxers and small breeds are reported to have a greater incidence of such adenomas. Because this results in **canine Cushing's disease** (**hypercortisolism**), it is discussed under Adrenal Cortex.

Aging dogs frequently develop nonfunctional pituitary tumors (**panhypopituitarism**), commonly cancerous. However, a number of other causes of reduced pituitary function are stroke (blood clots or broken blood vessels in the pituitary area), parasite invasion, nearby tumors that place pressure on the pituitary, or the results of injury due to trauma. Because so many endocrine glands (adrenal cortex, thyroid, etc.) may become secondarily involved, symptoms are quite varied. They may include depressed behavior, lack of coordinated movement, visual disturbance, loss of weight and muscle wasting, disturbances in water balance that result in dehydration (despite high water consumption), excessive urine excretion, and failure to remain housebroken. Note how general these symptoms are and how important it is to avoid overlooking many other causes of similar symptoms.

Corticotropin production may decrease following treatments with glucocorticoids. The cause may be interference with the normal feedback system that controls corticotropin synthesis. *This may complicate treating older dogs with corticosteroids, which are often used in arthritis and various inflammatory conditions.* See the discussion under Adrenal Cortex.

Growth hormone (GH), sometimes called **somatotropin**, acts on virtually every body tissue, stimulating protein synthesis in mammals of all ages and promoting growth in preadults. The hypothalamus controls growth hormone production in the anterior pituitary through somatostatin, which inhibits production, and growth hormone releasing hormone (GHRH), which stimulates production.

The action of GH on bone growth and maturation is indirect. The liver produces polypeptides called **somatomedins** in response to GH, and these act on the cells that are responsible for bone growth.

Increased blood plasma concentrations of amino acids, as after meat digestion, or decreased glucose, as during fasting, bring about growth hormone production. Its effects on fat and carbohydrate metabolism are interesting: **lipolysis** (fat breakdown) results in increased blood fatty acids and **glycogenolysis** (glycogen breakdown to glucose) is inhibited; thus, GH appears to have an anti-insulin effect.

Excess growth hormone caused by pituitary dysfunction in adult dogs, sometimes because of a functioning tumor, causes **acromegaly**. Acromegaly is age-related, with a mean onset at about 8.4 years of age. In this condition, bones become inappropriately thickened and features coarsen in appearance. The resulting changes in protein metabolism affect **connective tissue**, causing enlargement of the abdomen, excessive skin folds, and increased spaces between the teeth. **Gigantism** is the consequence of excess GH production in young dogs.

Some progesteronelike hormones are administered to suppress the estrous period in bitches. One, **medroxyprogesterone acetate**, has been shown to cause increased GH secretion and the symptoms of acromegaly. Effective treatment is to stop the drugs or remove the ovaries, if they are the source of excess progesterone.

Prolactin (PRL) is the anterior pituitary hormone needed by mammals for the production of milk by the mammary gland. Some studies show that it may influence male sexual attributes by promoting increased numbers of testosterone target cells, enhancing testosterone's effects.

THYROID GLAND

The thyroid gland is located in the neck or throat area near the **larynx** (voice box). It is common in dogs to find many accessory bits of thyroid tissue in many places between the larynx and the **diaphragm**. To say the least, this complicates thyroid surgery.

This gland produces two similar thyroid hormones and another very different one, **calcitonin**, which affects calcium metabolism (see under Parathyroid Glands, Vitamin D, and Calcitonin). The difference between the thyroid hormone molecules is that one contains three iodine atoms T_3 and the other contains four and is known as T_4 or **thyroxine**. (T_3) is much more potent; it has been shown to be lower in the serum of older men. The same appears to be the case in dogs.

Thyroid hormone acts on virtually all tissues; it raises the metabolic rate of cells. Additionally, thyroid hormone makes more glucose (blood sugar) available for energy metabolism, promotes the synthesis of proteins, influences several types of fat metabolism, and causes an increased heart rate.

Hypothyroidism (a deficiency in thyroid function) is the most commonly diagnosed thyroid disorder in dogs, with Doberman Pinschers and Golden Retrievers quite commonly affected. The production of thyroid hormone may be decreased following injury to thyroid tissue or the lack of iodine with which to make its hormone. One prominent thyroid condition in dogs, **lymphocytic thyroiditis**, may be inherited; it resembles **Hashimoto's disease** in humans. Considerable evidence supports an **autoimmune** (immune reaction against self) component in Hashimoto's disease and, perhaps, other hypothyroid conditions. The symptoms may include lack of energy, hair loss, skin thickening, decreased heart rate, and increased body weight. Of greater impact, hypothyroidism may be accompanied by muscle wasting, arthritis, liver malfunction, and the symptoms of **Addison's disease** (see under Adrenal Cortex).

Hyperthyroidism, rather uncommon in dogs, causes the opposite: increased heart rate, increased appetite and metabolism with accompanying weight loss, sleeplessness, vomiting, thirst, and diarrhea are observed. Muscular weakness and fatigue are often present.

Some thyroid malfunction may be related to the anterior pituitary's failure to produce thyrotropin. Also, several dietary substances (e.g., raw soybeans) may produce an enlarged thyroid called **goiter**. However, adequate dietary iodine usually reduces the effect of such goiter-producing substances. The possibility of autoimmune thyroid disease as a consequence of the use of modified live virus vaccines is an object of current studies.

Treatment of nonmalignant thyroid disease is well developed. The enlarged thyroid gland may be reduced by surgery or the administration of radioactive iodine. Also, antithyroid drugs such as propylthiouracil can be used to block excess thyroid hormone production. Hypothyroidism is relatively easy to control by giving sodium levothyroxin and similar drugs to replace the missing thyroid hormone.

GONADS

As discussed above, the gonads respond to the stimulus of gonadotropin from the anterior pituitary by producing steroid hormones. The term *estrogen* applies to one group of female hormones; estradiol is one of the most prominent individual estrogens. Testosterone is the primary male sex steroid. During part of the female's **estrous cycle**, and especially during pregnancy, progesterone (meaning "in favor of pregnancy") is produced. Excess progesterone may cause symptoms of acromegaly because of its secondary effect of increasing growth hormone production (see The Anterior Pituitary, above). The sex hormones will be described in more detail in the chapter The Reproductive System, where age-related changes will be presented.

ADRENAL CORTEX

The outer layer (cortex) of the **adrenal gland** differs significantly from the inner portion (medulla) of the same gland. The adrenal gland is actually two distinct glands; either the cortex or the medulla should always be specified for clarity of communication. The name *adrenal* derives from the prefix *ad-* (meaning "near" or "adjacent to") and a reference to the kidney, the *renal* organ, because the structure sits over the kidney in dogs.

The steroid hormones of the adrenal cortex belong to two classes. **Glucocorticoids** affect carbohydrate, fat, and protein metabolism. **Mineralocorticoids** influence mineral metabolism, especially sodium and potassium. A third steroid, **dehydroepiandrosterone** (DHEA), is currently receiving attention as a primary hormone.

Cortisol and **corticosterone** are glucocorticoids, and most cells of the body are their target. These hormones have **anti-inflammatory** action and are often used to suppress pain and swelling in parts of the body. Interestingly, the human **hippocampus**, a brain area important in memory, has glucocorticoid receptors that decrease in number with aging, a phenomenon needing more research.

Cortisol is a key hormone in the body's response to stress. Severe physical

---

The Second Messenger Mechanism

When a hormone (the *first messenger*) binds with a specific site on a cell's membrane, this causes the release of a *second messenger* from the membrane. This second messenger is usually derived from *adenosine triphosphate* (ATP). ATP is converted into *cyclic AMP*, adenosine monophosphate (cAMP), the second messenger itself.

Cyclic AMP may act to control immune activities, affect synthesis and release of hormones from the adrenal cortex, direct aspects of energy metabolism, mediate cell membrane permeability (the property of permitting passage of molecules), inhibit abnormal cellular growth, or alter synaptic potentials between neurons.

---

injury, extreme exercise, serious infection, extended exposure to major emotional distress or environmental extremes, and cardiovascular shock are associated with increased secretion of cortisol and a generalized activation of the sympathetic nervous system.

This reaction to stressors has been labeled the *fight-or-flight phenomenon* because it appears to prepare the individual to fight for survival or to flee from harm.

Cortisol stimulates the breakdown of protein to amino acids, which the liver converts to glucose. Small blood vessels become more responsive and blood pressure is better maintained because of increased cortisol. The sympathetic nervous system, especially via the hormones of the adrenal medulla, brings about an increase in blood glucose, increased fat breakdown products, decreased fatigue of the skeletal muscles, increased heart function, and increased blood pressure. The overall effect is that the stressed individual is initially prepared for efficient metabolism and a general tolerance of the changes the stress would otherwise cause.

Cushing's syndrome is a common endocrine disorder in dogs, and it is associated with overproduction of cortisol. It is age-related; the mean age for its occurrence is about 8.5 years. Poodles, Boxers, Boston Terriers, Dachshunds, and some Terrier breeds seem to be more commonly affected. It is most frequently caused by the pituitary gland producing excess corticotropin that stimulates the adrenal cortex.

Overgrowth of the adrenal cortex itself, especially noted in Poodles, results in increased cortisol production. About three-quarters of dogs with adrenal tumors are female. **Hypercortisolism** brings about increased blood glucose, general weakness with marked muscle wasting, thin and wrinkled skin, hair loss, unique mineral deposits in the skin, increased susceptibility to infection, poor wound healing, and hypertension. There is also an increased thirst, appetite, and frequency of urination. The resemblance between an aging animal and one with Cushing's syndrome has been noted for some time.

Treatment of individual dogs with glucocorticoids for medical reasons creates the risk of developing Cushing's disease. Frequent administration of glucocorticoids to treat inflammatory conditions is likely to lead to suppression of hypothalamic-pituitary control.

Aldosterone, the most prominent mineralocorticoid, promotes sodium re-absorption in the kidney. Retention of excess sodium and the water that associates with it contributes to an enlarged blood volume and **hypertension** (high blood pressure) in some humans. The problem in dogs may be less common. Many drugs have been designed to affect this control system by increasing sodium loss in the urine and causing water loss by increased urine output.

Addison's disease, most commonly seen in young and middle-aged dogs, is the consequence of general reduced function of the adrenal cortex. It is not as common as Cushing's disease. In most cases, the primary cause is atrophy of the adrenal cortex.

Dogs with Addison's disease lack conservation of sodium by the body and they excrete potassium. They may experience weight loss, low blood pressure, dehydration, general weakness, and even shock (failure to maintain sufficient blood pressure). The low blood concentration of glucocorticoids in Addison's disease allows blood glucose levels to fall when the dog is not eating (**hypoglycemia**), causes **anorexia** (loss of appetite), and seriously reduces the ability to tolerate stress.

Symptoms of Addison's disease can develop quickly in response to a rapid withdrawal of glucocorticoid therapy. This is a very dangerous disease that is capable of sudden changes. It should be aggressively treated by your veterinarian with hormone administration and infusions to reestablish salt and water balance.

ADRENAL MEDULLA

The medullary area of the adrenal gland is discussed at length in the chapter The Central Nervous System. Its role as part of the sympathetic nervous system is its primary function. It should be recalled that epinephrine and norepinephrine are the hormones of the adrenal medulla.

PARATHYROID GLANDS, VITAMIN D, AND CALCITONIN

The **parathyroid glands** are small masses of tissue embedded in the thyroid gland. The functions of their hormones are distinct from thyroid hormone functions. **Parathyroid hormone** (PTH), with vitamin D and **calcitonin** from the thyroid, controls calcium and phosphate metabolism.

The active form of vitamin D (**1,25-dihydroxyvitamin D**) is a steroid hormone. Active vitamin D is ordinarily the end product of several synthetic steps that begin with the effect of sunlight on a compound called **7-dehydrocholesterol** in the skin. Active vitamin D production takes place in the kidney with the aid of PTH. A healthy kidney adjusts the excretion of calcium and also is indirectly involved in the many actions of active vitamin D.

Hypercalcemia

Cancers are the most common causes of symptomatic **hypercalcemia** (high blood calcium) in dogs and humans. The tumors most frequently associated with hypercalcemia in dogs are **lymphosarcoma** and **adenocarcinoma**, often derived from **apocrine** glands surrounding the **anal sac**.

Functional tumors of the parathyroid gland may cause **hyperparathy-roidism** (excess production of PTH) with resultant hypercalcemia. About 25 percent of dogs with Addison's disease have high blood calcium levels.

As dangerous as treatment with corticosteroids may be in some instances, when a dog has lymphosarcoma their brief use seems justified in quickly lowering excessive blood calcium. Cortisol appropriately inhibits several of the factors that participate in bone breakdown.

Acute hypercalcemia can be treated in several other ways. Transfusion of salt solution (sodium chloride, NaCl) will expand the blood and body water volume and effectively dilute the calcium in the blood. It causes urinary excretion of calcium. This is usually a temporary measure. Ultimately, the cause of the hypercalcemia must be corrected. The drug furosemide promotes calcium excretion and may be a helpful adjunct to infusion of salt solution. Compounds called *diphosphonates* inhibit bone breakdown, thereby diminishing that source of calcium. Often used to treat other conditions, thiazide diuretics should *not* be used during hypercalcemia because they actually decrease the excretion of calcium by the kidney.

The heart is seriously threatened by an imbalance of calcium and other electrolytes in the blood. Death is near whenever the calcium level and its relationship to potassium becomes abnormal. An electrocardiogram may be useful in guiding the veterinarian's treatment.

Vitamin D is an excellent drug for the treatment of **hypoparathyroidism** (low parathyroid function). However, excess vitamin D may result in hypercalcemia with a risk of changes in bone and of calcium deposits in soft tissues such as the heart, kidney, and lung.

PANCREAS AND DIABETES

The pancreas is a mixed gland; it is both exocrine because it produces digestive products and endocrine because it produces hormones. The dog plays a significant role in our knowledge of the endocrine functions of the pancreas. The discovery of insulin and its effectiveness in controlling **diabetes** was first established by studies in the dog.

Diabetes is a very frequent endocrine disease in dogs. Most cases of diabetes are in dogs over five years old. Female dogs of many breeds and the Samoyed and Dachshund breeds are highly susceptible.

An inherited form of diabetes, which is most frequent in young dogs, is characterized by loss of the insulin-producing β-cells in the pancreas. It is called **Type I diabetes**, as it is in humans, and it has been frequently reported in the following breeds: Keeshond, Labrador Retriever, German Shepherd Dog, Standard Poodle, and mixed breeds. Because they lack pancreatic β-cells, these animals are clearly dependent on insulin.

The later onset type of diabetes (**Type II**) in dogs is more common. Humans with Type II diabetes often have abundant insulin production. They may control the disease with weight loss, exercise, and diet. The defect is that the body's cells do not adequately *respond* to insulin. In cases of mild diabetes in dogs, a diet low in carbohydrate and high in protein may be sufficient. However, in most cases, insulin injection is required, accompanied by small frequent meals of the appropriate kind.

In some cases, growth hormone excess can lead to diabetic symptoms. It appears to do so by bringing about resistance to insulin in the body's cells. Also, glucocorticoids can induce symptoms of diabetes. Veterinarians will be alert to this risk because hypercortisolism caused by adrenal cortex dysfunction or corticoid administration is common.

Insulin facilitates the movement of glucose across cell membranes; this is how it lowers blood sugar. Blood sugar is high in diabetic animals because glucose is not able to enter cells and be metabolized. Insulin enhances **glycogen** formation in the liver and skeletal muscles, increases amino acid levels in the blood, and promotes the formation of fat (**lipogenesis**).

When insufficient insulin prevents effective utilization of glucose for body energy, a shift to the use of fat occurs. **Ketoacids**, small 2-carbon fragments of fatty acids, are the products of fat breakdown. In excess, these shift the blood toward an acid composition. This condition (**acidosis**) *is a medical emergency and may quickly lead to fatality.*

Dogs with diabetes are now treated with injections of **protamine-zinc insulin** or the NPH form, replacing the insulin that the dog's own pancreas does not produce. Dedicated home care is needed for effective treatment. The urine of diabetics tends to have glucose in it because of the high blood levels. However, daily urine testing for glucose in dogs does not assure good control of the disease. A veterinarian can help establish other criteria for home care, which may include monitoring the dog's attitude, appetite, physical activity, water consumption, urinary continence, body weight, and urinary ketones. If on two or more consecutive days the signs change, or if a single instance of positive urine ketones is observed, the veterinarian should be called.

Future treatment may include implantation of β-cells from a donor, special insulin pumps, and the nasal administration of special forms of insulin. Obviously, these developments will be welcomed by dog owners as well as human diabetics.

Older dogs sometimes have pancreatic tumors, and usually they are malignant. The excess insulin produced by these functional tumors leads to muscle twitching, an unsteady gait, confusion, muscle weakness, and even unconsciousness. These tumors may sometimes be successfully removed.

Glucagon, a pancreatic hormone, increases glycogen breakdown (**glycogenolysis**) into glucose and fat breakdown (**lipolysis**), actions that are opposed to those of insulin.

Insulin and glucagon will be discussed again in connection with **intermediary metabolism** in the chapter Nutrition and Metabolism.

STOMACH AND INTESTINE

It is not common to think of the stomach and intestine as sources of hormones. Gastrin (from the stomach) and two intestinal hormones, **secretin** and **cholecystokinin** (CCK), were among the first hormones discovered. Evidence indicates that the brain is responsive to some of these, and emotions may influence their production.

Gastrin, a peptide hormone, is secreted by cells of the stomach wall in response to amino acids and peptides and following parasympathetic nerve stimulation. It reaches other **gastric** (stomach) cells via the blood, and it stimulates gastric glands to produce **hydrochloric acid** (HCl).

Cholecystokinin (CCK) and secretin act on the pancreas to stimulate secretion of enzymes and an alkaline solution that neutralizes acidic material from the stomach. In the intestine, CCK is produced when fat and products of protein digestion are present. CCK also promotes **bile** release by the **gallbladder**. This hormone may play an important role in control of appetite by signaling appetite control centers in the hypothalamus during the course of food digestion and absorption.

The hormone systems of the stomach and intestines appear to function well in young and old dogs. No evidence points to them as factors in disease or frequent malfunction.

THYMUS

Located under the **sternum** (breastbone) and near the heart, the **thymus** produces important immune cells and hormones. These are polypeptides called **thymosins**. These hormones are required for the competence of certain immune cells (see the chapter The Protective Role of the Immune System). The thymus gland undergoes a marked reduction in the number of its cells and overall size after puberty. By age forty in humans, thymosin levels begin to decrease. This loss of immune system function may contribute to aging. The role of thymosins is less well studied in dogs.

PROSTAGLANDINS

There are many variants among the **prostaglandins**, and it appears that all tissues produce them, rather than only a single gland. The biological life spans of these molecules are measured in seconds. One prostaglandin may have one action while another has the opposite. Examples are raising and lowering blood pressure or regulating local blood flow.

Some prostaglandins modulate nerve function by inhibiting impulse transmission and stopping the release of norepinephrine at sympathetic nerve endings. The pain-reducing (**analgesic**) effect of aspirin results from inhibiting the synthesis of certain prostaglandins. Others are involved in **immune** and **allergic** reactions. They also affect anti-inflammatory actions, inhibit blood platelet aggregation, and reduce blood clotting. Some regulate fat metabolism by inhibiting or counteracting the effects of hormones that promote fat breakdown.

The effects of prostaglandins on the reproductive system include destruction of the **corpus luteum** of the ovary and contraction of the uterine smooth muscle during the birth process. Various prostaglandins stimulate some exocrine and some endocrine glands.

All of these findings indicate the extensive involvement of these agents in physiological processes. There is, however, no current evidence of their involvement in aging.

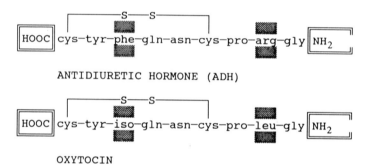

ANTIDIURETIC HORMONE (ADH)

OXYTOCIN

Similarity of ADH and Oxytocin Peptide hormones, such as antidiuretic hormone (ADH) and oxytocin, are formed by joining several amino acids. The type and order of amino acids determine the biological activity of the hormone. Three letter abbreviations stand for each amino acid. These two molecules are identical except for two of the nine amino acids.

7

The Gastrointestinal System: Intake and Digestion

THE **GASTROINTESTINAL SYSTEM** is responsible for ingestion, digestion, absorption, and excretion of food-related material. The gastrointestinal system starts with and includes the mouth (and its accessories, the teeth and salivary glands) and ends with the anus. Other important accessory organs are the liver and the exocrine portion of the pancreas.

The gastrointestinal tract may actually be viewed as part of the outer surface of the body because it is, in effect, continuous with the skin. It is a highly specialized system that deals with material taken from the environment and suitably processes it for subsequent entry into the body. Components of the immune system help prevent undesirable entry of infectious organisms. The **tonsils**, located near the beginning of the esophagus, are part of the **lymphoid system**. Many other components of the lymphoid system are located along the digestive tract, and an extensive drainage of lymph vessels exists. The saliva contains antibiotic substances, and the acidity within the stomach is also protective.

GENERAL ORGANIZATION

The divisions of the gastrointestinal system are the **mouth, esophagus, stomach, small intestine** (and its three parts: the **duodenum, jejunum,** and

ileum), **large intestine** (**colon**), **rectum**, and **anus**. Carnivores (meat eaters) such as dogs have shorter intestines than herbivores (plant eaters) because they do not need the extensive digestive structures required to digest plant matter.

The wall of the gastrointestinal tract has several layers. The innermost layer, the **mucosa**, is composed of epithelial cells that are often modified into glands that produce digestive enzymes. The cells making up this lining surface have the highest replacement rate of any in the body, with the possible exception of some white blood cells. They are replaced entirely every few days. In some areas, this layer also contains cells that produce hormones. **Sympathetic** nerve fibers innervate the mucosa.

The **submucosa** lies just beneath the mucosa and has connective tissue containing large blood vessels. The **muscularis** has two layers of smooth muscle. The inner layer is circular and the outer layer is longitudinal. This allows muscular movement to act on the digestive tract's contents. Local modification of the muscularis is found in the esophagus, stomach, and colon.

The nerves of the stomach, intestinal tract, and parts of the esophagus are both **intrinsic** (an internal network) and **extrinsic** (coming from the central nervous system). Generally, nervous system sympathetic activity inhibits gastrointestinal activity. The parasympathetic division excites gastrointestinal activity.

Mucus is universally produced by glands throughout the gastrointestinal tract. Not only does it lubricate and provide associated water as a solvent for ingested substances, but it is poorly digested. Thus, it serves as a coating to protect the mucosal surfaces from the system's own digestive enzymes.

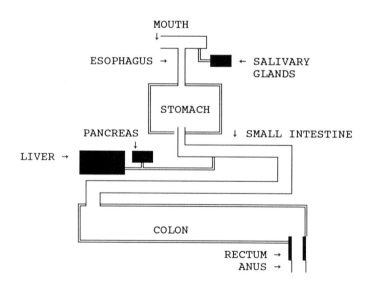

Anatomy of the Gastrointestinal Tract   The major parts of the gastrointestinal tract and the tissues and organs associated with it are illustrated.

THE MOUTH

The **teeth**, the **tongue**, the **mucosa surfaces** of the mouth, and the **salivary glands** are associated with the mouth.

The teeth are designed for tearing and chewing foodstuff. Dog teeth are typical of carnivores, but less so than the cat. The ability to tear food and to bite as if shearing is served by the design of the teeth.

It is generally known that puppies have a set of temporary teeth, **decidual teeth**, that are replaced by the **permanent teeth** of the adult. The average number of permanent teeth is forty-two, but this varies with breeds; the number of teeth expected in many breeds is specifically stated in their standards. Unfortunately, teeth are not always permanent. Teeth, themselves, may survive well; it is the supporting bone and the attachments that fail.

The tongue contains skeletal muscle and is under voluntary control. Also, its sensory capacity is well developed for touch and taste, the latter by virtue of **taste buds** on its surface. In humans, these receptors are known to be more or less specific for **sweet, sour, salt**, and **bitter**. Each type of receptor has a characteristic location on the tongue. Most substances are likely to stimulate more than one type of taste bud. Because dogs do not chew their food to any great degree, they may not use taste as much as odor in evaluating their food.

Salivary glands produce saliva that is either watery (**serous**) or **mucous** (contains **mucin**). Serous saliva contains an enzyme, **lysozyme**, which has **bactericidal** properties. The presence of lysozyme in saliva may explain why animals have a natural inclination to lick wounds.

Saliva also contains sodium and other minerals; substances such as steroid hormones are also present in saliva in concentrations similar to the same hormone levels in the blood. In humans, and probably dogs, white blood cells migrate from the blood between the teeth and the gums (the **gingiva**). Mucous saliva lubricates the surfaces of the mouth, making it easy to chew and form a portion of food into a mass (**bolus**) suitable for swallowing. Of course, the water of saliva serves as a solvent for soluble foodstuff.

Parasympathetic and sympathetic nerves control the salivary glands. A center in the brain stem mediates stimuli that affect salivary secretion. The presence of substances in the mouth, the thought of preferred food, and some odors bring about saliva production by nervous reflex. The normal production of a large amount of saliva daily demands good whole-body hydration, which sometimes does not occur in aged dogs.

Chewing

Dogs and other carnivores chew their food much less than humans. They tear food into small enough sizes to be swallowed and "bolt" the pieces. Chewing and swallowing are complex acts requiring a high degree of sensory and motor coordination. Chewing breaks food units into suitably small particles and mixes them with saliva. The act of swallowing takes place when a **bolus** (food mass) is tipped onto the back of the tongue where it stimulates receptors of the reflex. The coordination and progress of the act depends on a nerve center in the **medulla oblongata**. As the bolus begins to move into the dog's upper esophagus, the **epiglottis** closes over the **trachea** (windpipe), thus preventing food material from entering the trachea.

THE ESOPHAGUS

The esophagus has both circular and longitudinal muscle layers that generate wavelike contractions called **peristalsis**. Peristalsis moves the contents along the esophagus toward the stomach.

At the point where the esophagus joins the stomach there is a ring of muscle, a sphincter called the **cardia**. Normally, this helps isolate the stomach from the esophagus. When the peristaltic wave of the esophagus reaches the cardia, the sphincter relaxes and permits the bolus to enter the stomach.

THE STOMACH

An important role of the stomach is to store food. It is not widely appreciated that little digestion and almost no food absorption takes place in the stomach. After some processing, the material in the stomach is passed on in small portions to the small intestine without overwhelming the latter's digestive and absorptive abilities.

The strong **hydrochloric acid** (HCl) that is secreted in the stomach serves as a barrier to infection by killing many bacteria and viruses that are ingested with the food. Additionally, the acid environment is a good solvent for many substances in the food, and some digestive breakdown does begin here. The only enzyme secreted in the stomach is **pepsin**, a **protease**. Pepsin digests protein down to **polypeptides**; other enzymes split the peptides into **amino acids**.

The stomach produces a hormone, **gastrin**. It is released into the blood, reaching the glands of the stomach to stimulate HCl and enzyme production. Another hormone, produced in the duodenum of the small intestine in response to acid, is **gastric inhibitory peptide** (GIP). It inhibits the glands and muscles of the stomach, thus helping to protect the intestine from too rapid gastric emptying.

Mild contractions sweep over the stomach at intervals, mixing the contents but not creating the force necessary to send the material to the small intestine. In time, the digestive changes and the mixing of considerable water from the saliva and the **gastric** (stomach) secretions convert the stomach contents into a semiliquid mass that can pass into the small intestine. Then, periodically, powerful peristaltic contractions sweep toward the lower end of the stomach, which is separated from the small intestine by the **pyloric sphincter**. This sphincter does not freely open but does allow the passage of contents that are liquid enough and propelled by sufficient pressure from stomach peristalsis.

Control of a dog's gastric motility and secretion is both intrinsic and extrinsic. The extrinsic nerve supply of the stomach is through the autonomic nervous system.

Control of gastrointestinal activity is divided into three phases, the **cephalic phase**, which is mental, the **gastric phase**, and the **intestinal phase**. The sight, odor, or thought of food may initiate the cephalic phase. Salivation occurs, but this anticipation includes some gastric secretion as well. The famous experiments of Pavlov showed that ringing a bell whenever food was presented to dogs developed a conditioned reflex. Thereafter, ringing the bell alone initiated the cephalic phase responses.

Placing food in the mouth stimulates a more pronounced salivary and gastric response. The pancreas secretes digestive agents in response to this stimulus, too. Response to increased stomach contents and chemoreceptors for peptides in the food initiate the gastric phase. Centers in the medulla oblongata and the intrinsic neuron plexuses act to increase gastric secretion and movements. Gastrin participates in this phase.

The intestinal phase begins with the arrival of the acidic stomach contents to the small intestine. Acidity and fat in the contents stimulate reflex and hormone-induced slowing of gastric motility.

The stomach plays a unique role in the absorption of vitamin B_{12} (see the chapter Nutrition and Metabolism). It produces a protein known as **intrinsic factor** that combines with vitamin B_{12}, without which absorption will not occur. Absorption of the complex does not take place until it reaches the last portion of the small intestine, the ileum. Three conditions are necessary for vitamin B_{12} absorption: a dietary source of the vitamin, adequate intrinsic factor production by the stomach, and an effective absorption mechanism in the small intestine. Dogs rarely show trouble with this process.

THE SMALL INTESTINE, LIVER, AND PANCREAS

Almost all digestion and absorption of foodstuff takes place in the small intestine. It is divided into three segments: The duodenum is a short portion that follows the stomach, the jejunum is the middle segment, and the ileum is the last region.

The duodenum is the most dynamic portion of the small intestine. It receives acid stomach contents, generates and responds to neuron and hormone signals, and accepts **bile** from the liver and digestive aids from the pancreas. This begins the processes of digestion and absorption.

The dog's liver produces bile, storing it in the **gallbladder** until it is released following appropriate stimuli. The gallbladder is connected to the duodenum by the **bile duct**, which joins a similar duct from the pancreas just before reaching the intestine. A sphincter guards the neck of the gallbladder. Relaxation of the sphincter and contraction of the gallbladder is initiated by a hormone, **cholecystokinin** (CCK). Endocrine cells in the duodenal mucosa produce CCK in response to the presence of fat and acid.

Bile contains **bile salts** (sometimes called **bile acids**); they are synthesized from cholesterol, and cholesterol itself is secreted into bile. Bile salts are fat **emulsifiers**, breaking fat into smaller units that enable enzymes to have greater access to them. Considerable amounts of the secreted bile salts and cholesterol are reabsorbed in the intestine.

A pancreatic fluid rich in **bicarbonates** neutralizes the acid reaching the duodenum. This alkaline product follows stimulation of the pancreas by the hormone **secretin**, which is produced by cells in the duodenal wall. Secretin was the first hormone discovered.

Proteases of the pancreas split proteins to **dipeptides**. Proteases of the intestine complete the job by splitting the dipeptides into **amino acids**. Pancreatic **amylase** breaks down **polysaccharides** such as starch. These are not further reduced in size to **monosaccharides** (glucose, fructose, and galactose) by this enzyme. Final carbohydrate digestion is carried out by the intestinal enzymes **maltase** and **lactase**. Pancreatic **lipases** split triglycerides (**triacylglycerols**) into **glycerin** and **fatty acids**. More details are in the chapter Nutrition and Metabolism.

Amino acids and monosaccharides are absorbed by the intestine and delivered directly to the liver via the blood vessels of the **hepatic** (liver) **portal system**. Under this arrangement, blood from the capillaries of the intestine goes into the **portal vein** and enters a special circulation in the liver. The pattern of blood vessels in the liver allows an intimate percolation of the blood, so that liver cells have access to the substances right after they are absorbed. The liver processes much of the material (e.g., making glycogen from glucose, making plasma proteins from amino acids), and it detects and detoxifies many unwanted molecules that were absorbed.

Iron absorption is unique. Ordinarily, iron is quite toxic, and the dog's body manages a large amount of iron by absorbing and transporting it with special mechanisms. Various tissues (intestine, liver, spleen, bone marrow) store iron in a complex with protein called **ferritin** (see the chapter Nutrition and Metabolism).

Although researchers have presented theories based on participation of ferritin and transferrin to explain iron absorption, it is still unclear exactly how the mechanism works. In any case, iron absorption is controlled by the iron status of the individual; if a dog is iron deficient, a greater proportion of a test dose of iron will be absorbed.

Calcium also has a special absorption system. Calcium is transported across mucosal cells by combining with a specific **calcium-binding protein**. Active vitamin D, as a hormone (see the chapters The Endocrine System, Nutrition and Metabolism, and The Urinary System), is required for producing calcium-binding protein. Calcium in the diet may be the specific activator for its production.

THE LARGE INTESTINE, RECTUM, AND ANUS

Digestion is not a function of the large intestine. However, slight and specific absorption takes place here. Water is absorbed, helping to form the appropriate texture of **feces**. Excess water reabsorption results in too firm a stool and **constipation** occurs. Maintaining adequate water intake and ingestion of sufficient water-holding fiber are important ways to rectify this problem. Sodium is absorbed from the colon, but potassium is secreted. During **diarrhea**, considerable potassium loss may occur.

A large and normal population of bacteria inhabits the colon. These organisms are able to convert material, such as fiber, into nutrients for themselves. Vitamin K and some of the B vitamins are produced by these bacteria and absorbed from the colon. Much bacterial metabolism yields gaseous carbon dioxide, which is normally passed as **flatus** via the anus. The carbon dioxide in flatus is odorless. A large proportion of the feces consists of dead and living bacteria. The usual color of the feces is largely caused by the bile pigments in it.

The rectum and anus end the gastrointestinal tract. Normally, the rectum remains empty except when especially powerful muscular contractions propel material into it, stimulating that part of the defecation reflex that opens the **anal sphincter** and allows the rectum to expel the feces. The anal sphincter is divided into one portion that is involuntary smooth muscle and another part that is skeletal muscle that can be controlled voluntarily. Without the latter, dogs could not become housebroken.

AGING AND THE GASTROINTESTINAL SYSTEM

It is difficult to distinguish which gastrointestinal changes are caused by age and which are caused by diseases and medications. However, the epithelial lining of the system seems to become somewhat thinned by a slower turnover rate of its cells. Barring disease, abuse, or dietary neglect, the gastrointestinal system typically functions well in healthy elderly dogs.

MOUTH

A loss of taste buds on the tongue brings about reduction in the ability to taste, at least in humans. This loss reduces appetite and nutritional intake.

A lack of saliva is serious. Usually it can be traced to disease or the effects of many medications, especially those that influence the function of the autonomic nervous system.

The loss of teeth is not a certainty of aging. Much can be done to protect against tooth loss. The dental profession often makes the statement that ''teeth are meant to last a lifetime.'' See the discussion below for more on oral disease and dental care.

ESOPHAGUS AND STOMACH

Old esophagus (**presbyesophagus**) describes the motor malfunction of swallowing in which the esophagus and the cardia are not coordinated. In humans, this may fail when the cardia is not tightly closed and acid stomach contents may regurgitate into the esophagus. Also, failure of the cardia to open properly may result in considerable discomfort. Because these conditions are not associated with acute symptoms that indicate a threat to the animal, dogs may have them more often than reported.

Inflammation of the gastric mucosa is associated with wasting of its cells (**atrophic gastritis**) and occurs in very old humans. This causes a reduction of gastric juice production. Again, dogs may have less trouble than humans, and very old dogs may have so many other complications that atrophic gastritis is overlooked. A more easily digested diet may still be prudent for the very old dog.

PANCREAS AND LIVER

The pancreas and liver, if uninjured and uninfected, generally function well in old age in dogs and humans. The pancreas responds to stimulation by producing a normal volume of pancreatic juice and the bicarbonate content is undiminished. Pancreatic amylase and trypsin are somewhat reduced in the elderly, but not so much so that protein and carbohydrate digestion is inadequate. A similar reduction in lipase is of no concern unless fat intake is above reasonable levels.

In elderly dogs, bile secretion probably remains unchanged. Unless disease is present, liver function tests can be expected to be in the normal range in a healthy elderly dog. Plasma **bilirubin**, one of the pigments of degraded **hemoglobin**, is removed by the liver and secreted via the bile. Its plasma concentration ordinarily does not exceed normal, but it may if the ability of the liver to excrete it has been lost.

The liver is unusual among the tissues of mammals because it has the power to regenerate after part of it is removed. This property diminishes until adulthood in humans. It *does not continue* to diminish as aging progresses.

Ordinarily, the liver inactivates chemical toxins that have been absorbed or produced by the body. Also, the liver metabolizes many drugs, usually converting them to substances that are more easily excreted by the kidney.

SMALL INTESTINE

Diminished fat absorption may be related to a reduction in lipase production by the pancreas. In old age, reduced calcium absorption may occur in dogs; malabsorption of calcium is present in most very old humans. Elderly humans also absorb iron less adequately, and the same is true for vitamins B_1 and B_{12}. In otherwise healthy dogs on good diets, such reductions in vitamin and iron absorption should not present problems.

The blood flow through the intestinal mucosa is reduced in the aged. However, absorption appears to remain adequate.

LARGE INTESTINE

Although constipation and **diverticulosis** (inflammation of pouches in the intestinal wall) are common complaints of elderly humans, they are not normal accompaniments of aging in humans or dogs maintained on appropriate diets. The older dog's diet should be monitored for necessary adjustments. A dog should not be subjected to laxatives unless a veterinarian finds a specific medical reason for doing so.

DISEASES OF THE GASTROINTESTINAL SYSTEM

Diseases of the gastrointestinal system are common and distressful to elderly dogs. Some conditions are merely uncomfortable. Others are either life-threatening or point to dangerous diseases in other tissues. Endocrine or neuron tumors may affect gastrointestinal function.

MOUTH AND LOSS OF TEETH

Few things are more distressing in the elderly dog than loss of teeth. *It is not an aging process; it is a disease that can be prevented.*

The first step is to carefully examine the dog's mouth at regular intervals so that oral health can be ascertained. Concerns about a dog's oral health should be discussed with a veterinarian.

The roots of teeth are very vulnerable in their sockets of bone, and the area of the gums (**gingiva**) is subject to infection. Chewing stimulates a strengthening of all components. A diet of relatively hard substance is preferred over soft foods. Even dogs seem to understand this need by their fondness of chewing on bones and leather items.

Soft diets and those rich in sweets encourage the growth of bacteria that are responsible for the deposit of **plaque**, which is central to the formation of mineralized deposits of **tartar** (**calculus**). Bacterial growth causes deterioration of the connections between the gums and the teeth. Pockets of infection are formed under the gum line, and more serious infection undermines the attachment between tooth surface and gums. When this infection proceeds into the area where the roots of the teeth are anchored in their sockets, support is lost and the teeth become loose. This stage is full-blown **periodontal disease** and is quite difficult to treat satisfactorily. The dog owner's responsibilities include providing proper diet in terms of both nutritional composition and texture—and following the veterinarian's instructions on supplemental oral care.

Unlike humans, dogs do not often have cavities in teeth (**caries**). However, their activities may cause broken teeth, as well as other injuries to the mouth.

Firm **oral tumors** should be taken seriously because most of them are malignant. Exceptions are tumors originating from gingival (gum) tissue and the nonmalignant mouth tumor called a **ranula**. This is a cyst of the **salivary duct** of the **submaxillary gland**. An aberrant growth of gum tissue should receive veterinary attention because it may interfere with actions of the mouth and may be bruised. The ranula, which causes blockage of a salivary gland's duct, is not common. Neither of these is necessarily age-related. However, malignancies are more common with age, so any growths in the mouths of older dogs should be appraised by a veterinarian.

Old dogs may show bacterial infection of the lips by a lesion where the hair and nonhaired areas of the lips meet. The infection may be caused by injury, but may also be related to deficiencies of B vitamins, allergies, and mange. The owner should attempt to determine the cause (running in weeds, for example) and control it. If home treatment is not clearly effective, see a veterinarian. Similarly, dogs with pendulous lips have skin folds on the lower lips that easily become infected (**lip fold pyoderma**) and may be noted by the foul odor from the mouth. Locate and cleanse the area and use the medication recommended by your veterinarian.

If your older dog has bad breath, a great many causes must be considered. **Stomatitis** means inflammation of the mouth. **Vincent's stomatitis (trench mouth)** is caused by some of the microorganisms normally found in the mouth. Some changes in the lining of the mouth (mucosa) allow these common micro-organisms to infect the mucosa. It can spread, for example, causing pneumonia. Vincent's stomatitis, which may include parts of the tongue, may lead to **gangrenous stomatitis**. A severe deficiency of the B vitamins can cause this as well. This is a severe condition requiring prompt veterinary care. Oral ulcers characterize **ulcerative stomatitis** and may occur in debilitated old dogs suffering from a number of other serious diseases. Malnutrition, general disease, and unsanitary environments may contribute to **granular stomatitis**, a chronic condition that requires a veterinarian to properly diagnose and treat it. Sometimes, ulcerative stomatitis (**mycotic stomatitis**) may be caused by a common yeast organism called *Candida albicans*. When inflammation involves the tongue it is referred to as **glossitis**; inflammation of the gums is called **gingivitis**.

Dry mouth (**xerostomia**) may occur in older dogs for a number of reasons. Among the conditions that contribute to dry mouth in the aged are certain drugs, dehydration caused by the use of **antidiuretic** medicines and insufficient water intake, and mouth breathing because of nasal obstruction or respiratory distress. Drugs that cause a reduction in saliva formation include atropine and sodium pentobarbital.

Excessive drooling (**ptyalism**) may be traced to a number of poisons and irritants; foreign bodies, missing teeth, and other injuries to the mouth; infectious diseases, including rabies and distemper; salivary cysts; and, especially, nervous responses related to fear. Because rabies may be accompanied by ptyalism, it is imperative that a veterinarian be consulted.

ESOPHAGUS

Difficulty in swallowing (**dysphagia**) may occur in dogs because of organic diseases, some of which are common to age. This difficulty is associated with problems such as neuromuscular dysfunctions, cancer of the wall of the esophagus, inflammation caused by the parasitic worm *Spirocerca lupi* in the wall of the esophagus, chronic use of or exposure to certain insecticides, or a nerve-muscle condition called **myasthenia gravis**. Any condition that affects muscular coordination elsewhere (e.g., movement or vocalization) may also interfere with the muscles of swallowing.

STOMACH AND SMALL INTESTINE

Gastritis means an inflammation of the stomach and **enteritis** means an inflammation of the small intestine; either may be chronic or acute. A great many infectious microorganisms and parasites may be the cause, as well as foreign objects, ingestion of irritating substances, and allergies. Some systemic diseases, such as distemper, coronavirus, parvovirus, and hepatitis (liver inflammation), cause inflammation of the small intestine. Furthermore, enteritis often involves the stomach (**gastroenteritis**) or the colon (**enterocolitis**). The sophisticated techniques needed for precise diagnosis of these conditions demand veterinary care.

Canine hemorrhagic gastroenteritis is a serious disease in mature dogs. It has a rapid onset with bloody diarrhea from intestinal bleeding, collapse of the animal, and death if not treated. The cause is not known, but there may be a relationship to bacteria-produced toxins. Small-sized breeds seem more susceptible. Attention by a veterinarian is imperative.

Coronavirus (**canine coronaviral gastroenteritis**) is a highly contagious disease. It seems to be restricted to dogs, foxes, and coyotes. Dogs at any age may become infected, showing the initial symptoms of diarrhea and vomiting. The stool often has a notable odor and may contain blood. Since it is quite contagious, the disease may spread quickly when numbers of dogs are in contact with one another, as in kennels. Otherwise healthy adult dogs given antibiotics and supplemented for loss of fluids may fare well. A killed vaccine available from your veterinarian will protect against this disease.

Parvovirus (**canine parvoviral infection**), an enteritis, occasionally occurs in older dogs, but it is primarily a disease of the very young and has symptoms similar to coronavirus.

The numerous parasites that may cause gastroenteritis and enterocolitis include large **roundworms** (**ascaridoid nematodes**), **hookworms** (*Ancylostoma caninum*), and **tapeworms** (various **cestodes**). Because they are large and are passed in the feces, roundworms may be noted by a dog's owner. Careful examination of the feces may reveal eggs or adult forms of other intestinal parasites, but the average owner lacks the skill to do an effective diagnosis. Now that a number of relatively safe medications for some intestinal parasites are available, these infestations can be controlled.

However, beware of the idea behind the statement that a dog has been "wormed." That only means that some kind of medication, at some dosage, has been administered; whether it was an appropriate and effective treatment is not established. Only a veterinarian can effectively differentiate between these conditions and suggest or provide adequate treatment.

Gastric dilation and torsion (bloat) initially involves extreme distension of the stomach by air, secretions, or food. At some point the stomach rotates (**volvulus**), making normal emptying impossible. The enlarged stomach and the twisting at the gastric-intestinal junction interrupts blood flow to the tissues involved. Considerable damage to these tissues and other abdominal organs (e.g., the spleen) takes place. **Shock** (vascular collapse) may occur.

Although seen in dogs of the smaller breeds, large and giant dogs are more susceptible, especially those with deep chests. This condition is a true and urgent medical emergency. A stomach tube passed down the throat may succeed in allowing the stomach contents to escape, providing temporary relief. Stabilizing the cardiovascular function is needed to prevent shock. Surgery is required to restore the anatomical relationship between the stomach and intestine. Subsequent care is often difficult, with shock and heart malfunction threatening for some time.

PANCREAS

Pancreatic cancer may involve the exocrine cells of the pancreas or the pancreatic duct. These cancers (**adenocarcinomas**) are usually seen in older dogs. The mean frequency is nearly eleven years of age. Liver disease, including liver cancer, may accompany pancreatic cancer. Loss of body weight, loss of appetite, signs of liver malfunction, and vomiting are such general symptoms that the veterinarian may find diagnosis difficult. Treatment with surgery is unlikely to be helpful because loss of the pancreas is a serious matter in its own right, especially when added to the trauma of surgery.

Acute pancreatic necrosis appears to be more common in dogs than in other domestic animals. The death of cells (**necrosis**) is simply the effect of a number of assaults on the tissue. Physical trauma to the pancreas, occlusion of the pancreatic duct that leads from the pancreas to the intestine, and reflux of bile or intestinal contents into the pancreas via the pancreatic duct are among the causes. Another possible cause is a failure of local blood flow to the pancreas. This allows a release of the gland's powerful digestive enzymes, which act on its own cells. Working dogs or those in good physical condition are not likely candidates, but middle-aged and old dogs that are overweight and eat a diet containing considerable fat are predisposed to pancreatic necrosis. Abdominal pain, mild or severe, and vomiting are symptoms. However, they are too general to diagnose the condition without various blood tests that the veterinarian can perform.

LIVER AND GALLBLADDER

One of the functions of the liver is to excrete, via the bile, pigments from hemoglobin following the normal turnover (destruction and replacement) of red blood cells. Liver malfunction at any age may cause **jaundiced** (a yellow discoloration of areas such as the white region of the eyes), reflecting the high level of bile pigment accumulated in the blood. However, obstruction of the bile duct, more common in the aged, also prevents excretion of bile pigments.

Two important consequences of diminished liver function are that blood levels of poisons (toxins) remain high, and drugs in doses suitable for younger dogs may be excessive for older dogs because they are *not processed and removed* as rapidly in the elderly.

The liver has the ability to regenerate its mass to some extent. Also, it ordinarily has a large functional reserve, which may be reduced in an aging dog. For these reasons, the liver must often be considerably damaged before signs of **hepatitis** (liver inflammation) are evident. The liver relates to the functions of so many other tissues and organs that the symptoms observed may make evaluation or diagnosis very difficult for a veterinarian. Liver function may be altered by parasites (liver flukes, tapeworm cysts, etc.), infections (viral, bacterial, fungal), toxins (from certain plants, organic and inorganic poisons, and even vitamin D overdose), nutritional deficiencies (cobalt, vitamin E, selenium), certain endocrine and metabolic disorders (e.g., Cushing's syndrome), congestive heart failure, and bile duct obstruction.

Infectious canine hepatitis (ICH) is a contagious disease in dogs and related carnivores. It is caused by a **canine adenovirus**, which can be shed with feces, saliva, and urine of infected animals. The immune cells of the intestine and the tonsils become infected, as does the liver. Other involved tissues include the kidneys, spleen, and lungs.

Even after recovery, dogs shed the virus in their urine for a number of months. ICH may be mild in some cases but fatal in others, especially very young animals. Many of the liver's metabolic roles are affected. Blood clotting is impaired, reflecting the fact that the liver is the source of certain elements essential for blood clotting. A modified live-virus vaccine is available and is commonly administered when puppies are vaccinated against distemper.

Leptospirosis, caused by any of several **leptospiral organisms**, results from contact of the skin or lining of the mouth with contaminated urine, food, or water. It has been called **canine typhus**, **infectious jaundice**, or **Stuttgart disease**. Often, the most conspicuous symptom is **hemorrhagic gastroenteritis**, but it is described here because of liver involvement. Dogs of all ages become infected, especially males. Old dogs have less reserve to withstand the extensive organ dysfunction, which may include the liver, the kidney, and the heart. Despite the dramatic illness of infected dogs, recovery is likely if a veterinarian's attention is prompt and thorough. Humans are susceptible to the leptospiral organisms that infect domestic animals and require appropriate protection from dogs that have leptospirosis.

Malabsorption Syndromes

Malabsorption syndromes may be caused by failure to digest foods because of lack of pancreatic digestive enzymes, bile production or release, or lack of intestinal enzymes. A wide range of infectious organisms and parasites in the small intestine have been suggested as responsible for malabsorption. In cases associated with lack of bile, failure to effectively absorb fat products results in fatty diarrhea (**steatorrhea**) as a symptom.

Weight loss accompanies the loss of nutritional substances. Low protein nutrition may lead to low blood plasma proteins and result in leakage of fluid into tissue spaces (**edema**). Inefficient absorption of vitamin B_{12} and iron may lead to lack of sufficient blood hemoglobin (**anemia**). If vitamin K is not well absorbed, the liver is unable to manufacture the substances required for proper blood coagulation. A malabsorption syndrome is a complex condition, requiring a veterinarian for diagnosis and treatment.

COLON (LARGE INTESTINE), RECTUM, AND ANUS

Colitis (inflammation of the colon's lining) has been discussed to some extent with enteritis. Straining to defecate and frequent bowel movements are symptoms. Perhaps the most common cause is parasite infestation, especially by whipworms and hookworms.

A large number of factors may be related to **colon impaction** (constipation). Inactivity, often characterizing the elderly, can contribute to constipation. Other causes include cancer of the colon, painful anal conditions that inhibit defecation, inappropriate diet (e.g., feeding excess bones or low residue foods), obstruction of the bowel or the anal opening by foreign objects, and deformation of the colon (e.g., rectal diverticulum or hernia in the perianal area).

Paralysis caused by spinal injury or disease can contribute to constipation, and enlargement of the prostate gland may press on the rectal area enough to impede fecal movement. Because some of these factors are life-threatening (e.g., cancer, lodged foreign objects), a veterinarian should be consulted rather than relying on traditional methods to relieve simple constipation by the use of mineral oil, enemas, etc. The use of medications such as anticholinergics and morphine derivatives (e.g., codeine) inhibit gut motility and allow the fecal dehydration that leads to constipation.

Serious at times, constipation alone is not generally the health threat that many other gastrointestinal conditions can justly claim. The popular notion that serious bacterial toxins are absorbed from the colon (**autointoxication**) is not substantiated by research. Archaic views promote this idea of gastrointestinal function.

Rectal prolapse is the protrusion of the rectum through the anus; only the mucosal layer may be evident or all of the rectal wall may protrude to some degree. Boston Terriers appear prone to this condition because of a genetic predisposition. Many diseases have been associated with rectal prolapse. Both sexes and all ages may suffer from it. The deterioration of health in the aged dog, especially prostatic enlargement, cancer of the colon and rectum, and straining from constipation, may contribute to rectal prolapse. If severe and long-standing, surgery is commonly required.

Perineal hernia (a herniation in an area near the anus) is reported to be more common in Welsh Corgis and Boston Terriers, particularly in uncastrated male dogs six to eight years old. In some way, hormones of the male may play a role, especially via hormone-caused prostatic enlargement. Most of the hernias contain a rectal deviation. Straining to defecate contributes to the condition. Difficult bowel movements and **flatulence** (passing rectal gas) are common signs. Perineal hernias must be surgically repaired by a veterinarian.

Strictures (a narrowing of a tubular structure) of the rectal or anorectal areas are not frequent, except in German Shepherd Dogs, Beagles, and Poodles. Scar tissue from wounds or infections are primary causes. Bowel emptying is compromised and veterinary care is required.

Older male dogs that have not been castrated, especially Beagles, Bull-dogs, Cocker Spaniels, and Samoyeds, have cancer near the anus (**perianal adenoma**) with some frequency. This condition is actually a skin-related cancer because the **perianal gland** is a modified sebaceous gland in the anal area. The cancers in this tissue may be of various types. Although much rarer and not primary to the perianal gland, several other cancers may occur in the perianal area.

Older dogs, especially over seven years, may experience **perianal fistula**, which is a deep ulcerlike tract draining into the anal area. The material produced is especially malodorous. Its causes are unknown, but the infection that is as-sociated with it may spread to other tissues in the area with serious conse-quences. Surgery is usually required.

Anal sac disease (disease of the **anal gland**) is the most common disease found in the anal area; smaller breeds are at greater risk. Because these sacs release a substance that tags the feces with identifying odors, their contents are partially expelled by the pressure of defecation of feces of normal texture. Soft stools and inadequate muscle pressure may cause the sac to retain its contents, resulting in inflammation. The discomfort leads a dog to pay attention to the anal area by licking and biting, it may be unable to comfortably sit, and it often drags the anus against the floor or other surface. A veterinarian can express the gland and determine the cause of the dog's difficulty, as well as determine if there may be a cancer.

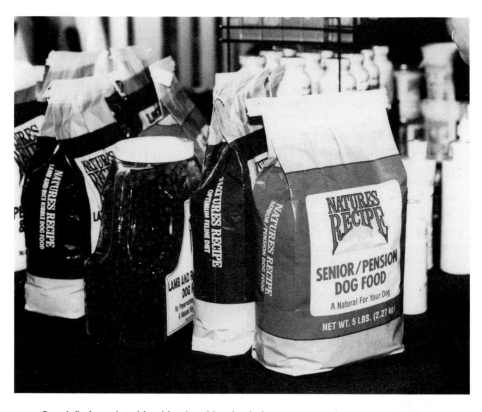

Specially formulated food for the older dog helps ensure maximum use of nutrients.

8

Nutrition and Metabolism: Processing and Functions of Foodstuff

NUTRITION, so obviously connected with well-being, has been a key in efforts to modify human life span. With domestication of animals, especially companion dogs, it is not surprising that owners relate some of these concerns to their pets.

The role of exercise in nutritional balance will be discussed in the chapter The Cardiovascular System. The type and amount of activity an animal experiences interacts with its metabolism and its nutrient needs. The primary effect of metabolism is energy production rather than the smaller, but important, amount of metabolism involved in growth and repair of tissue.

Old animals are less able to repair tissue injury or regulate body temperature. Excess fat and simple sugars (e.g., sucrose or glucose) in the diets of humans and dogs in the United States constitute malnourishment as surely as deficits in calcium, iron, or vitamins. However, dogs may metabolize fats somewhat better than humans. This has been recognized by several dog food manufacturers who prepare diets to match the needs of the aged.

NUTRITION AND METABOLISM

DIGESTION AND ABSORPTION

As discussed in the chapter The Gastrointestinal System, ingested foods must be altered before they can be absorbed. Proteins must be broken down into amino acids, and carbohydrates must be split to monosaccharides. These fundamental units are absorbed from the intestine by active transport systems.

Fats are not dependent upon active transport mechanisms. For efficient absorption, they must be emulsified and broken down to fatty acids. Vitamin B_{12} is clearly dependent upon controlled absorption. Some minerals, such as calcium and iron, have specific absorption mechanisms. Once absorbed, **assimilation** takes place, which refers to the body's use of the absorbed material.

Proteins

An enormous variety of protein molecules can be assembled from amino acids. These proteins play a major role in the body as plasma proteins, antibodies, enzymes, structural and functional elements of cells, connective tissue (e.g., **collagen**), and some hormones. Protein complexes include **glycoproteins** (protein-carbohydrate combinations), some of which are good lubricants (e.g., **mucus**), and **lipoproteins** (lipids combined with proteins), some of which represent fat in transport via the blood.

After absorption, amino acids may be considered a pool from which cellular metabolism draws the ones needed for any particular synthesis of **amines**, **peptides**, **polypeptides**, or protein molecules.

The dog is unable to significantly store amino acids. A blood plasma protein, **albumin**, will be broken down when the reserve of amino acids is low. **Edema** (swelling of tissue) may be caused by low blood plasma albumin. Albumin is important for its ability to hold water in the vascular system. However, skeletal muscle is probably a more important source for emergency supplies of amino acids. Muscle wasting is a characteristic of protein-deficient animals.

When amino acids are present in abundance they may serve as fuel for the energy metabolism of cells or may be converted to fat. The liver and kidney form **urea** from released amine groups and excrete it.

Dogs may be able to efficiently handle slightly larger protein intakes than humans. Commercial dog food with 22 to 28 percent of average quality protein is common. However, a diet with protein comprising 14 to 21 percent by dry weight seems a suitable recommendation for older dogs, according to some authorities. Age-related reduction in liver and kidney function limits the ability of elderly animals to tolerate very large amounts of protein.

When carbohydrate stores are low, amino acids may be converted to glucose. This process is called **gluconeogenesis** (creation of new glucose) and takes place during starvation or fasting, thereby maintaining a blood glucose level suitable for nervous system energy metabolism. Some amino acids can be derived from others, but several of the twenty amino acids the body needs must be ingested in the diet. These are referred to as **essential amino acids**, an unfortunate designation because all twenty amino acids are essential. The term simply refers to the fact that it is essential for these to be acquired from the diet. Dogs on appropriate commercial diets are not at significant risk of essential amino acid deficiency, *but* a diet from the human table might present that risk.

Some authorities feel that low protein diets may prevent kidney disease and failure, but this remains controversial. The evidence is overwhelming that it is beneficial to lower dietary protein after kidney disease has developed. Of course, your veterinarian should provide accurate diagnosis and guide you in selecting the best diet for older dogs with kidney disease.

Hormone Influences on Protein Metabolism

Growth hormone (GH) is the most abundant hormone produced by the anterior pituitary gland. It is quite important for functions other than growth during development. It mobilizes fat as an energy source, but it reduces muscle's use of glucose.

Insulin, known to be involved in glucose metabolism, also has many actions resembling growth hormone. It increases transport of amino acids across cell membranes, increases the DNA transcription process, and speeds up protein synthesis.

Male sex hormones (e.g., **testosterone**) are significantly related to protein metabolism in skeletal muscle. Development of muscle mass and strength depend on these hormones. Some loss of strength and muscle mass in natural aging may be related to the progressive reduction of testosterone.

A group of growth-promoting peptides affects normal and abnormal cell growth. One, the widely distributed **nerve growth factor** is similar to insulin in structure and function. Another is **epidermal growth factor**. It stimulates growth in **epidermal tissue** (outer skin layer) by its influence on mRNA (messenger RNA) production. **Fibroblast growth factor** has been found in the pituitary gland and brain, and experimental studies indicate that it is involved in some tissue regeneration (e.g., regeneration of limbs in salamanders). These substances have been studied in many species and their functions are probably typical in dogs.

Thyroxine, the hormone of the thyroid gland, is essential for normal growth and metabolism. A deficiency in young animals also produces inadequate brain and mental development. Lack of thyroxine results in excessive production and deposition of mucoprotein (a cell-to-cell cement). This produces a condition referred to as **myxedema** (see the chapter The Endocrine System).

Glucocorticoids (e.g., the steroids cortisol and cortisone) affect liver by accelerating the processes of gluconeogenesis, protein synthesis, and breakdown of amino acids.

Fats (Lipids)

The main representatives of fats in the body are the **triacylglycerols** (also known as **triglycerides** or **neutral fats**—storage fats), **phospholipids** (fats of membranes, fats in transport complexes, etc.), and **cholesterol** (the precursor of steroid hormones and an important constituent of cell membranes).

Triacylglycerols are made of three fatty acids attached to a molecule of **glycerol**. Fatty acids are considered **saturated** if they contain all of the hydrogen ions that can be attached. Otherwise, they are called **unsaturated** fatty acids. Some fatty acids are modified to hormonelike **prostaglandins** (see the chapter The Endocrine System).

Cholesterol is handled somewhat uniquely. As a lipoprotein complex, it attaches to specific receptors of liver cells. Within liver cells, cholesterol is used in making **bile salts**, which act to emulsify fats in the intestine. Cholesterol is actually eliminated via bile as cholesterol or in an altered form (**bile acids**). Although some of this material is reabsorbed, the net effect is a loss of cholesterol; excretion by the liver is the only known way to eliminate cholesterol.

For a dog to use fatty acids for energy, they must be broken down. Fats yield over twice as much energy per gram as carbohydrates or proteins. Fats are not only an efficient energy source, they comprise the greatest amount of readily available stored energy. However, the nervous system can only use glucose, and glucose will be used initially by muscle during exercise.

Glucagon, growth hormone, **epinephrine**, and **corticotropin** are hormones (see the chapter The Endocrine System) that bring about the release of fatty acids from fat stores, a process called **lipolysis**. On the other hand, insulin promotes the synthesis of triacylglycerols.

If a dog lacks insulin, cells are unable to effectively synthesize fatty acids and triacylglycerols. The result is a high blood level of fatty acids and glycerol. General fat deposits become depleted, but the liver is still able to store fats excessively.

In the absence of insulin, the liver also produces **ketone bodies** as well as **acetone** (see the chapter The Endocrine System). If the **ketosis** (high blood level of ketone bodies) is great enough, it may result in an **acidosis** (shift of the blood to a more acid state), *threatening coma and death*. A similar situation obtains during starvation. In obese dogs, the switch from glucose to fat metabolism may accumulate enough ketone bodies to be quite dangerous.

Studies on some species (especially rodents and, perhaps, humans) have demonstrated that a diet high in fat reduces life span, and skin and mammary tumors appear earlier in life. Increased fat intake in rodents is associated with a decrease in immunity and an increase in autoimmune diseases. Certain fat sources differ in their effects; for example, a fatty acid from cottonseed oil increases mammary tumors in mice.

There is reason to believe that various species of animals differ considerably in their ability to tolerate high fat diets. Dogs and "pure" carnivores (e.g., cats) are probably more tolerant than humans and herbivores (plant eaters). Dogs may tolerate diets with fat as high as 50 percent, although 6 to 8 percent by dry weight is adequate. However, obesity is a threat to the best health in all species, and aging compounds the problem.

Dietary fat requirements of older dogs probably do not differ much from younger ones. It has been suggested that the fat content in the diet should be somewhat greater than 10 percent based on dry weight, with a minimum of 5 percent. The essential fatty acid in the dog's diet is **linoleic acid**. This is easily obtained from a normal mixed diet and its lack is rarely the cause of a disease. Fat-soluble vitamins (A, D, E, and K) require fat absorption to be absorbed themselves. If a dog has intestinal, liver, or pancreatic disease, it may have problems with fat absorption.

Carbohydrates

Humans have a greater ability than dogs to digest uncooked starches and cereals. Therefore, such foods should be *well cooked* to accommodate a dog's digestive system. Other than that, dogs digest and use carbohydrates for energy about as effectively as humans. Dogs may have up to 60 percent of their calories supplied by carbohydrates.

Some dogs lack the enzyme (**lactase**) to digest milk sugar (**lactose**). Diarrhea and intestinal cramps are symptoms of excess dietary lactose.

Much of the dog's energy comes from carbohydrates. However, glucose and other carbohydrates have other metabolic and structural functions. Examples are **heparin**, an **anticoagulant** (inhibits blood coagulation) found particularly in the liver, **hyaluronic acid** found throughout the body as intercellular cement, and **glucosamine**, a glucose molecule associated with **mucin**.

Glucose, as well as amino acids and lipids, contribute to the production of **adenosine triphosphate** (ATP), a molecule which stores the energy needed for metabolism. This is accomplished by the **Krebs cycle**, a series of chemical reactions by which one molecule of glucose yields thirty-six to thirty-eight molecules of ATP.

Vitamins

Vitamins are nutritional substances required in very small amounts to enhance the functions of enzymes. They are classified according to their solubility in water or fats. These properties affect the intestine's ability to absorb most of them. Vitamins A, D, E, and K are fat-soluble; the remainder will dissolve in water.

As a dog ages, food intake may be less, although it still meets its reduced requirements for calories. However, this may result in a deficiency of other nutrients, such as vitamins. If your veterinarian suggests vitamin supplements, it has been suggested that A, B_1, B_6, B_{12}, and E are the ones most likely needed.

Fat-Soluble Vitamins

Vitamin A is fat-soluble in its primary form as **retinol**. However, a water-soluble compound, **beta-carotene**, may be converted to retinol. It is found in animal products such as liver and milk. Beta-carotene comes from many yellow and dark green vegetables.

Liver storage of vitamin A and its dietary availability make vitamin A sufficient in old dogs with normally good nutrition. Retinol is toxic in excess amounts, but beta-carotene is much better tolerated; its conversion to retinol is limited to need.

As retinol, vitamin A is incorporated into photopigments (see the chapter Awareness of the Environment and the Special Senses) that enable the eye to see in dim light. Night blindness results from vitamin A deficiency. Epithelial tissues appear to need vitamin A for their maintenance; the cornea of the eye may develop opacities when vitamin A is lacking. In toxic amounts, vitamin A causes dry skin, hair loss, and liver damage.

Vitamin D, needed for normal calcium absorption and use, does not enter into metabolic activities in the way the other vitamins do, but behaves more like a hormone (see the chapters The Endocrine System and The Urinary System). Excess vitamin D (**hypervitaminosis D**) initially causes bone calcification, but later on it causes bone demineralization; calcification in joints, kidneys, heart muscle, and lungs may also occur.

A **vitamin E** deficiency is difficult to induce. Large amounts of vitamin E have been shown to have no harmful effect—but no advantages either. When this vitamin is lacking, red blood cells are more fragile, and urinary excretion of creatinine (indicating muscle breakdown) is increased.

Vitamin E is abundant in foods having high polyunsaturated fatty acids. The same intake seems adequate for young and old dogs; it is easily supplied by good diets. Extra vitamin E will not enhance sexual attributes in any way despite some lore to that effect.

The **vitamin K** needs of older dogs is usually met because adequate amounts are synthesized by normal bacteria in their intestines. As with vitamin E, large doses of vitamin K seem relatively harmless. Difficulty in absorbing fat may result in a shortage of vitamin K. Prolonged use of antibiotics may alter the intestinal bacteria that synthesize much of the vitamin K needed. Vitamin K is required for liver synthesis of proteins involved in blood coagulation. Lack of vitamin K results in easy bruising and abnormal bleeding.

Water-Soluble Vitamins

The water-soluble vitamin **thiamin** (**vitamin B_1**) was the first vitamin discovered. Humans on a diet of polished rice developed a condition called **beriberi**, which could be cured by thiamin, a substance found in rice husks. Thiamin deficiency is characterized by a reduced appetite and weight loss, convulsions and other central nervous systems signs, muscular atrophy (wasting), peripheral **neuritis** (inflammation of peripheral nerves), and, occasionally, paralysis.

Riboflavin (**vitamin B₂**) deficiency is difficult to produce in dogs, but, if present, it may cause decreased body temperature, decreased respiratory rate, unsteady gait (**ataxia**), and even death. A veterinarian can test for riboflavin status with a special test—a measure of **glutathione reductase**.

Nicotinamide (**niacinamide**), sometimes called **vitamin B₃,** is another water-soluble B vitamin; it has no association with the nicotine of tobacco. It is also called **niacin** or **nicotinic acid**. Some microorganisms can make nicotinamide from the amino acid tryptophan, but dogs must ingest it. A deficiency gives rise to **canine pellagra** (**black tongue disease**), a condition characterized by diarrhea, **dermatitis** (skin inflammation), and altered mental function. It is now rarely seen because of commercial diets with proper protein ingredients, instead of diets with a high content of corn.

Vitamin B₆ affects function of the nervous system in both deficiency and excess. It is certainly not one of the water-soluble vitamins that are harmlessly excreted as sometimes claimed. Dermatitis also develops when B₆ is lacking.

Biotin is needed for amino acid and protein metabolism. With deficiency, muscle pain and fatigue develops, and a poor appetite complicates its lack.

Folic acid (**folacin**) received its name after its isolation from spinach leaves (**folium** means "leaf"). A deficiency in dogs may cause **glossitis** (inflammation of the tongue), a low white blood cell count, and an anemia characterized by a few large red blood cells, each containing more than usual hemoglobin (**macrocytic hyperchromic anemia**). In this case, it resembles the effect of vitamin B₁₂ deficiency. Severe folic acid deficiency leads to mental impairment that is reversed upon restoring the vitamin intake to normal.

Vitamin B₁₂ is one of the most potent biological compounds, the daily need being extremely small. Present only in foods of animal origin, it is easily available to all but strict vegetarians who must be attentive to its need; dogs should not be maintained on a vegetarian diet. **Pernicious anemia** (a **macrocytic** anemia) and problems related to nucleic acid synthesis may occur because of a deficiency of vitamin B₁₂. Lack of vitamin B₁₂ may also result in neurological disturbances and impaired peripheral sensations. When lack is severe and long-lasting, paralysis may develop.

Vitamin B₁₂ is absorbed only in the last portion of the small intestine (the **ileum**) and only after it has combined with a mucoprotein from the stomach called **intrinsic factor** (see the chapter The Gastrointestinal System). A genetic abnormality that results in the lack of intrinsic factor production or the disease **ileitis** (inflammation of the ileum) may result in malabsorption. The vitamin must then be administered by injection. It is stored in the liver, making daily injection unnecessary. Reduced production of intrinsic factor in an elderly dog may be a result of atrophy (wasting) of the stomach mucosa.

Vitamin C (**ascorbic acid**) in a small amount is required to prevent the deficiency symptoms of **scurvy** in humans: fragile blood vessel walls, poor wound healing, and impaired bone metabolism. This vitamin is important in collagen synthesis and maintenance of the material that cements cells together. Dogs manufacture the vitamin C they need, and dietary supplements are questionable. It has been claimed that stress and extreme activity may call for supplements of vitamin C, but this is unconfirmed.

Minerals

Calcium and **iron** are minerals abundant in the skeleton and red blood cells. Other minerals such as sodium, potassium, and phosphorus are also plentiful in the body. Some minerals play vital roles in relatively small amounts. Yet all, including iron and calcium, are significant in functions where small amounts are the rule.

A small amount of iron is important in the energy-producing metabolism of the Krebs cycle. Calcium, besides being a component of bone, is required for blood clotting, muscle contraction, and nerve and muscle excitability.

Sodium is one of the major electrolytes of the dog's body. It is important for the polarization of nerve and muscle membranes (see the chapter The Excitable Tissues). Its osmotic ability to hold water makes it crucial to the fluids of the body, especially the blood volume and consequent blood pressure. The amount of sodium in a well-chosen diet for dogs is quite adequate.

Excess intake of sodium, as well as excess protein and phosphorus, is undesirable because it may cause kidney damage. It has been claimed that from 59 percent to greater than 85 percent of dogs older than five years have kidney disease to some degree. **Hypertension** (high blood pressure) is present in the majority of dogs with kidney failure, and this is caused, in part, by excessive retention of sodium and water. Congestive heart failure and edema may also be evident.

Elimination of excess dietary sodium, protein, and phosphorus has been shown to be beneficial to many dogs with kidney disease. Owners should not wait until these clinical conditions threaten the health and life of their dogs. Avoiding dietary excesses throughout life is a reasonable course to follow, especially because kidney disease is a leading cause of death in dogs.

Potassium, is the major intracellular electrolyte and is often involved in the same functions for which sodium is vital. Also, its relationship with calcium is quite important, because they have opposite effects on excitable tissue. Calcium in excess results in hyperexcitability with **tetany** (sustained contraction) of muscles. Potassium excess inhibits excitable tissue and can be lethal as a result of the failure of cardiac muscle activity. Potassium needs are well met by good commercial diets for dogs, and potassium supplements should be given only under veterinary supervision because of the serious effects of an overdose.

Phosphorus is a critical part, with calcium, of the compound that constitutes bone. In smaller amounts it is a part of ATP, the primary energy form for metabolism.

Iodine metabolism has been discussed in connection with its only significant biological role, as part of the thyroid hormones (see the chapter The Endocrine System).

Magnesium activates a number of enzymes and is important in normal nerve and muscle function. About two-thirds of the body's magnesium is in bone. Prolonged diarrhea may deplete it and dietary deficiency may occur. Its lack is associated with depression, weakness, and increased irritability.

Copper is critical to the enzymes that produce **hemoglobin**. It also is a part of **melanin**, the pigment that is present in dark skin. Copper deficiency is rare in dogs. Excess copper may cause copper deposits in some tissues and result in injury.

Zinc is a component of several enzymes. One of them is **carboxypeptidase**, an important digestive enzyme. **Carbonic anhydrase** is a zinc-containing enzyme that is essential for the blood's ability to transport CO_2. In an elderly dog, the lack of adequate zinc may account for impaired wound healing, poor hair growth, and loss of taste and appetite.

Dogs with cancer often have plasma zinc levels lower than normal. When given zinc supplements, they seem to have improved appetites. Furthermore, lack of adequate zinc in cancer patients may diminish immune system effectiveness and this impairs natural anticancer defenses.

Selenium is essential, but it is quite toxic in excess. It is a part of a compound that protects membranes of cells from damage by peroxides. Its antioxidant role puts it in a class with vitamin E.

Chromium is widely distributed in the environment. One of its roles is related to tissue response to insulin, and a deficiency results in poor removal and use of blood glucose. Although inefficient removal of blood glucose is common in the aged, it may be caused by many factors other than low chromium.

Fluorine is normally a constituent of teeth and bones. In adequate amounts it provides protection against dental caries (cavities). However, unlike humans, dogs have few caries.

Manganese activates some enzymes and aids the formation of urea. Lack of sufficient manganese may result in poor growth, anemia, bone changes, and impaired central nervous system function.

Cobalt is an essential component of vitamin B_{12}.

Vanadium is known to be essential, but its role is unclear.

Molybdenum is an essential component for some enzymes. It does compete with copper absorption and either one in excess may interfere with the other.

Silicon (the primary component in sand and glass) is an extremely abundant element. It is required for the calcification of bone. It is present in connective tissue and may participate in cross-linking on collagen molecules.

Iron Metabolism

Iron, the most abundant heavy metal in the body, is quite toxic. It is easily converted to **ferric hydroxide**, which is able to kill mucosa cells of the stomach and intestine. Iron pills are next to aspirin as a cause of the accidental poisoning death of children, and dogs might also be attracted to the shiny red pills if they are not kept out of reach.

No mechanism for controlled iron excretion exists as there is for calcium, sodium, potassium, etc. Therefore, except for incidental loss of iron by **hemorrhage** (blood loss) and cell **desquamation** (shedding of cells), once it has entered the body, it is recycled for various metabolic uses.

Iron deficiency anemia caused by lack of dietary iron is not common. In dogs, iron deficiency anemia may result from lack of gastric hydrochloric acid (**achlorhydria**), dietary substances that compete with iron absorption, impairment of the intestinal mucosa, and greatly increased iron loss from hemorrhage.

Certain parasites, especially hookworms, may be key factors in anemia. The seriousness of the causes of anemia makes it unwise to treat the symptoms without a veterinarian's advice. Anemia may result from factors other than iron deficiency, e.g., vitamin B_{12} deficiency or bone marrow damage.

Calcium Metabolism

The anatomy and physiology of bone is presented in the chapter The Skeleton and Skeletal Muscles. **Osteoarthritis** and other bone and joint diseases are also discussed there.

The appropriate way to examine calcium nutrition (as well as many other nutrients) is to measure intake and excretion. It should then be determined at what point there is a balance for nongrowing individuals or a **positive balance** for those who are growing. A **negative balance** exists when an individual experiences a net calcium loss.

The following are some of the more important factors that affect calcium and bone metabolism:

1. *The amount of ingested calcium and its form.* Calcium is not absorbed freely; it is absorbed partly by diffusion, reflecting its concentration in the intestine, and by an active transport system that is dependent upon active vitamin D for the synthesis of an intestinal calcium transport protein. The transport system may be defective even though calcium is abundant. Lack of hydrochloric acid in the stomach (achlorhydria) is an occasional age-related condition that can affect calcium absorption.
2. *The availability of active vitamin D.* As described in the chapter The Endocrine System, vitamin D in an active form may be considered a steroid hormone produced by the kidney. Adequate absorption of calcium requires active vitamin D.
3. *Protein intake.* It is often not appreciated that excess protein in the diet may significantly contribute to a negative calcium balance. The excess does so by increasing the excretion of calcium in the urine. One study of humans revealed that doubling protein intake increased calcium excretion 50 percent. The protein metabolism of dogs may significantly differ from that in humans, and dietary protein may have less effect on their calcium balance.

4. *Dietary fiber*. Research has shown that dietary fiber may influence calcium absorption by binding with it. Also, the intestine's opportunity to absorb calcium (and some other substances) may be reduced because of rapid intestinal transit time and dilution by water in the bulk material. Reasonable fiber intakes should not be of concern. The findings from research in humans may need modification when applied to dogs.

5. *Dietary phosphorus and magnesium*. A major portion of skeletal calcium exists bound with phosphorus, making adequate phosphorus in the diet important. Magnesium is another important but much smaller component of bone. It is recognized that appropriate phosphorus intake reduces urinary loss of calcium. Phosphorus is abundant in meat, bone meal, and many other foods. Unfortunately, some dog owners are so concerned about "good bone" in their animals that they administer excessive calcium and other minerals. Actually, an imbalance between dietary calcium, phosphorus, and magnesium may be created and cause the very conditions they seek to avoid.

6. *Dietary sodium*. The chapter The Urinary System deals with kidney function in detail. However, it is relevant to mention here that the ability of the kidney to conserve both sodium and calcium resides partly in a transport system common to both. Thus, excess sodium competes with the kidney function that retains calcium, resulting in increased calcium loss by urination.

7. *Drug effects*. The caffeine in tea, coffee, and cola drinks increases calcium in urine and digestive juices. It does not appear to affect absorption. The effect is small, but it may become significant. It is hard to imagine conditions in which dogs might consume excessive caffeine.

Food Restriction

Gerontologists report that *the only procedure known to significantly extend life span is calorie reduction*, assuming the diet is of high quality. Early interpretation took into account that maturity was delayed and even bone growth was retarded. However, smaller food restrictions without such severe effects have been shown to be effective in prolonging life. A most important experiment showed that rats on identical diets had life spans directly related to the amount of food they chose not to eat; *those that ate less, lived longer*.

Food restriction is effective in extending life span even when started after maturity has been reached. This indicates that delayed maturity is not responsible for extended life span. Animals in these food restriction studies had fewer age-related changes and diseases than those allowed free access to food.

Some gerontologists have raised the issue that by restricting their food intake, rodents are returned to a condition that more closely resembles their evolutionary heritage and their state in the wild. Some think that this observation is pertinent to modern human life in affluent societies and the life-style our dogs share.

Much more knowledge is needed before investigators pass a sound recommendation on to the public about dietary restriction for themselves or their pets.

Fiber

Fiber is defined as any nonabsorbable, nonnutritive material in foodstuff. This definition means that fiber is found in many chemical forms and may be expected to have a number of physical and chemical properties. An image of "fibrous" material such as **brans**, the coatings of grain seeds, comes to mind. Less familiar are the abundant forms of fiber that have the properties of **gels** and **gums**.

Excess dietary fiber has negative consequences, especially in an elderly animal with lower nutritional intake. Negative balances of iron, calcium, and magnesium have been observed in humans on very high fiber diets. **Flatulence** (intestinal gas) may be substantial on some high fiber diets.

Good diets for dogs have various types of fiber in them. Carnivores, with their shorter intestinal tracts, are less prepared to digest the types of food that humans may seek to provide fiber.

Dogs, especially older ones, do not need and may not be benefited by fiber levels as high as recommended for humans. One recommendation is that dogs should consume less than 7 percent fiber by dry weight. When weight reduction is required, fiber is useful because it provides bulk and replaces food calories. Moderate increases in dietary fiber may be indicated for old dogs with **diabetes mellitus**, **colitis** (inflammation of the colon), obesity, and constipation. Increased dietary fiber has been claimed to lower insulin requirements in diabetic dogs.

NUTRITIONAL PROBLEMS AND DISEASES

CANCER, DIET, AND METABOLISM

Cancer is more common in older dogs. Body weight loss is common and this is often reflected in blood elevations of free fatty acids and lipoproteins. The metabolism of fat, protein, and carbohydrate is altered in various ways in dogs with cancer. Loss of muscle mass is among the changes seen in protein metabolism. Carbohydrate metabolism is altered, as is sometimes seen in the insulin resistance that is typical of some diabetics. Dogs with cancer often show low plasma zinc levels, and zinc supplements may increase appetite and immune performance.

Cancer therapy, while of greatest importance, should not overlook attention to improved nutrition. Indeed, better nutrition may enhance the effectiveness of the therapy in several ways. Diets that support growth and reproduction may be appropriate, and the basic energy requirement of dogs with cancer may be as much as three times greater than usual.

OBESITY

The most common nutritional disease in dogs and cats (and humans?) *is obesity.* This is defined as a weight 15 percent greater than ideal. In dogs, obesity is more common than all other diet-related diseases combined. In a recent survey, it was determined that over 30 percent of dogs beyond five to seven years of age were obese. Age is a predisposing factor in obesity, and spayed females seem most susceptible. Beagles and Dachshunds have been identified as breeds prone to marked obesity. Of course, rapid weight reduction is uncomfortable and unwise. The **basal energy requirement** (BER) of your dog can be calculated by your veterinarian for a suitable weight loss program.

DIABETES MELLITUS

It has been pointed out (see the chapter The Endocrine System) that dogs commonly have **Type II diabetes**. Increasing insulin by injection is more often required in diabetic dogs than in humans, but sometimes effective control follows a reasonable exercise program, weight reduction, and restriction of intake of simple sugars. Even in nondiabetic animals, intake of simple sugars may result in undesirable blood sugar variations. Because simple sugars are so quickly absorbed, blood glucose levels may rapidly exceed normal and stimulate a marked secretion of insulin. Insulin may then drop blood glucose to below normal, a condition called **reactive hypoglycemia**. Furthermore, insulin is important for the metabolism of amino acids and fats; inducing high levels of insulin will disturb other areas of metabolism.

Caloric needs are reduced in the elderly dog. Eating refined simple sugars, which provide only calories, leaves little food to provide all remaining nutrients, including vitamins and minerals. The result is either a dietary deficiency or obesity if more food is eaten to meet these needs.

GLUCOSE METABOLISM

In aged individuals, a delayed reaction to glucose ingestion occurs; i.e., blood glucose does not return to normal as readily. The delayed reaction indicates that the aged metabolism has less ability to deal with glucose. The **glucose tolerance test** is much more likely to be abnormal in inactive dogs. The glucose intolerance of aging does not seem related to the reduction in lean body mass. Generalized undernutrition may play a role. This further suggests that care to avoid excess simple sugars is advisable.

Diabetics suffer a number of alterations in various tissues. Impaired sensation, damage to blood vessels in the kidney and eye, cataracts, and other tissue injuries that resemble age-related changes develop in diabetics. Collagen is affected in skin, blood vessel walls, and elsewhere; DNA injury occurs; and the properties of proteins in the eye lens are altered.

9

The Cardiovascular System: Function of the Heart and Blood Vessels

---

CARDIOVASCULAR MECHANICS

The heart and blood are responsible for giving warm-blooded animals a high, stable metabolic rate. This metabolism requires a cardiovascular system that will meet an enormous need for oxygen and carbon dioxide exchange. The cardiovascular circulation is a closed circuit under high pressure, and its smallest elements (the **capillaries**) are in intimate association with all cells.

The vascular system transports the blood through the lungs to receive oxygen and expel carbon dioxide, through the kidneys to modify the blood's composition, through the intestine and liver where foods and other chemicals are processed, and to the skin facilitating heat loss or retention. Cells in the various tissues of the body are supported by an ideal fluid environment provided by the blood.

ORGANIZATION OF THE CARDIOVASCULAR SYSTEM

The heart is actually two muscular masses: a relatively thin-walled **atrial muscle** and a powerful thick-walled **ventricular muscle**. Chambers within each

93

muscle are subdivided into two compartments with partitions. The **atrial** compartments are reservoirs for the blood returning to the heart. The ventricular muscle is a powerful two-chambered pump.

When the ventricular muscle contracts, blood (the **stroke volume**) is pushed into the two arteries leading from the right and left ventricular chambers. Blood is pumped to the lungs from the **right ventricle** by the pulmonary artery. Blood is carried from the **left ventricle** by the **aorta** to all other parts of the body.

At the beginning of each of these major arteries, one-way valves (**semilunar valves**, so-called because of their half-moon shape) prevent blood from leaking back into the chambers when the ventricular muscle relaxes. Additional one-way valves between the atrial and ventricular chambers (**atrio-ventricular— A-V valves**) are closed by the rising ventricular pressure. These A-V valves prevent blood from being forced back into the atrial reservoirs. The movement of blood through the lungs to the left atrial chamber constitutes the **pulmonary circuit**. The greater **systemic circuit** begins with the blood leaving the left ventricle through the **aorta** and ends when it returns to the right atrium.

Large arteries are lined with epithelial cells that form the **intima**. In addition to the fibrous protein **elastin**, the artery walls have layers of smooth muscle cells and an outer layer of connective tissue. Large arteries are particularly elastic; they are able to store energy in the form of blood pressure. As they divide into smaller arteries, and finally into **arterioles** (smallest arteries), elasticity is less prominent. The muscular walls of the arterioles, however, are especially important because they determine the variable diameter of these vessels and, thus, the **peripheral resistance** to blood flow.

One way to view **capillaries** is to consider them as arterioles from which

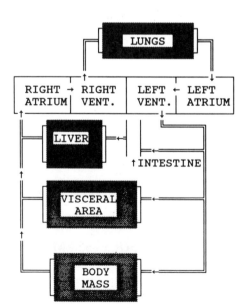

Diagram of Cardiovascular System
This is a diagram of the cardiovascular system. It demonstrates the flow of blood through the heart, lungs, and other tissues of the body. The blood's special path through the vessels of the intestine and liver is shown.

all layers of their walls have been removed except the intima. Such a thin wall (the intima only) is expedient because it is across the capillary wall that exchange of substances takes place between the blood and the **interstitial fluid** that surrounds cells.

Capillaries join together to form **venules**, which, in turn, become the **veins** that return the systemic blood to the right atrium. Venules and veins are less muscular than arteries and more able to relax and accommodate the volume of blood they receive. Instead of storing pressure, which is extremely low when compared with that in arteries, veins store the greatest part of the blood volume. After emptying into the right ventricle, blood is sent through the lungs to start the circulatory cycle over again.

The pulmonary circulation handles the same volume of blood per minute as the greater systemic circulation, but at a much lower pressure—about 15 mm Hg (millimeters of mercury) mean pressure, compared with 100 mm Hg in the aorta. The capillaries of the lungs are larger in diameter and the distance through this circuit is shorter. Because gas exchange is a rapid process, slow blood flow through lung capillaries is not particularly important.

HEART (CARDIAC) FUNCTION

The two muscle masses of the heart (atrial and ventricular) are separated by a connective tissue layer that anchors the two arteries (pulmonary and aorta) and their semilunar valves, as well as the larger valves (A-V valves) that prevent backward flow during ventricular **systole** (contraction). The closures of these valves are responsible for the "heart sounds," which are phonetically described as *lub-dup*. The first sound (*lub*), longer and of lower frequency, is caused by the closure of the A-V valves as the sudden ventricular contraction raises pressure above that in the atria and forces them closed.

During systole, as the pressure in the ventricles increases, the semilunar valves are forced open; this allows ventricular ejection of blood into the arteries. As systole subsides, ventricular pressure falls below arterial pressure and the semilunar valves are abruptly closed as the arterial blood pushes back against them. The semilunar valves are smaller and the vibration attending their closure is of higher pitch and briefer duration, creating the sound *dup*.

The continued fall in ventricular pressure as it relaxes results in a pressure below that in the atria. This allows the blood in the atria to gently push the A-V valves open and ventricular filling rapidly begins as the stored blood enters them.

The heart muscle has an inherent rhythm. It does not need signals from external nerves for the electrical activity that results in contraction. The only nerves to the heart are from the **autonomic nervous system**. **Sympathetic** nerves increase the rate and force of contraction, and **parasympathetic** nerves do the opposite.

A small bit of tissue that polarizes and depolarizes at a regular rate is located in the wall of the right atrium and serves as the pacemaker of the heart.

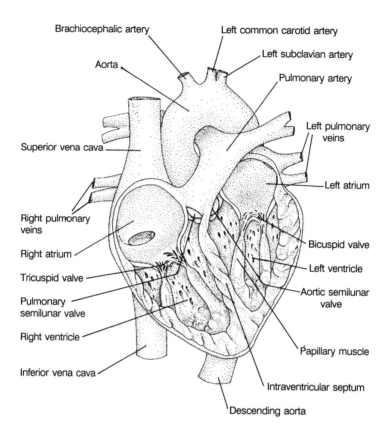

Typical Mammalian Heart The four-chambered heart serves the pulmonary and systemic circulatory pathways. Direction of flow is controlled by semilunar valves in the arteries. Large A-V valves direct blood from the atria to the ventricles. When the ventricles relax, the semilunar valves close and prevent blood from flowing back into the ventricles; closure of the A-V valves prevents blood from entering the atria during ventricular contraction.

This is called the **sino-atrial** (S-A) **node**. It is the point at which the heartbeat is ordinarily initiated. Other parts of the heart muscle (**myocardium**) and conducting system are also able to generate an electrical impulse, but at a slower rate. These sites generally remain inactive as long as the faster S-A node functions well.

In the wall of the right atrium is another specialized tissue mass, the **artrio-ventricular** (A-V) **node**. The impulse pauses here before going to the ventricular.

Impulses bridge the gap between the atria and ventricles by following a bundle of special conducting tissue, the **bundle of His**. The impulse is then distributed over the rest of the ventricle. The action potential activates the ventricular muscle from apex to base. The contraction "squeezes" the blood toward the area where the main arteries leave the ventricular chambers.

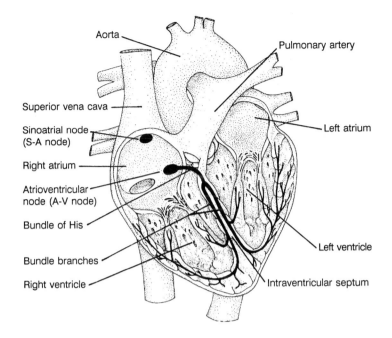

Aorta

Pulmonary artery

Superior vena cava

Sinoatrial node (S-A node)

Left atrium

Right atrium

Atrioventricular node (A-V node)

Bundle of His

Bundle branches

Right ventricle

Left ventricle

Intraventricular septum

The Heart's Electrical Conduction System   The impulse (action potential) that initiates heart muscle contraction is rapidly distributed throughout the heart muscle. The heart's pacemaker is the S-A node. The A-V node sends impulses to the ventricles, which then contract. These contractions pump blood into the arteries.

The myocardium differs from skeletal muscle in its metabolism. It ordinarily requires oxygen, whereas skeletal muscle is capable of considerable metabolism without oxygen. The heart's primary energy source comes from free fatty acids; it uses glucose less than does skeletal muscle.

Sodium ions are important for the **membrane potential** of cells. Calcium and potassium are also vital to impulse conduction. Calcium, in excess, produces a state of **hyperexcitability** and may prevent adequate relaxation of the myocardium. Potassium excess inhibits myocardial contraction and is also deadly.

The Electrocardiogram

The **electrocardiogram** (the ECG; EKG is an older term) is a record of the electrical activity accompanying the depolarization and repolarization of the atria, ventricles, and special conducting tissue of the heart (see the chapter The Excitable Tissues). The ECG record is made by placing **electrodes** (contacts) on the skin, thus in contact with the fluid of the body, and recording the electrical fields affecting the electrodes. No changes in the ECG will detect aging.

CARDIAC OUTPUT

Heart Rate

The **cardiac output** is measured in ml/min (milliliters per minute) and is an expression of the effectiveness of the pump. The frequency of heartbeat (**heart rate** in beats per minute) multiplied by the amount of blood ejected during each beat (**stroke volume** in milliliters) is used to calculate the cardiac output.

An average dog's cardiac output is 180 ml/kg/min (milliliters/kilogram of body weight/minute) during rest. It can increase five to eight times that value during exercise. In dogs that are physically well conditioned, the resting heart rate is lower than usual, as it is in human athletes, but they maintain normal cardiac output because of a greater stroke volume.

The heart rate is affected by the autonomic nervous system; the sympathetic division increases heart rate and the parasympathetic division decreases it. **Epinephrine** and **norepinephrine** from the **adrenal medulla** produce effects similar to sympathetic nerves. An increase in blood temperature and heart temperature increases the heart rate. Lower temperature has the opposite effect. Lowering of the temperature is used to quiet the heart during heart surgery.

Stroke Volume

Stroke volume has more complex elements than heart rate. The amount of blood in a ventricle's chamber at the end of diastole depends on ventricular filling. The duration of **diastole** is certainly a factor, but the **venous** return from the rest of the body has a major effect on filling. Stroke volume is influenced markedly by the amount of blood found in the ventricle at the end of contraction, reflecting the adequacy of emptying.

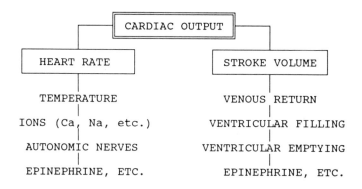

Factors in Cardiac Output This diagram illustrates important factors relating to cardiac output (CO). Significant factors that influence heart rate and stroke volume are also listed.

Modest overfilling stretches the myocardium and enhances its force of contraction, an advantage during exercise. The sympathetic division of the autonomic nervous system promotes a greater muscle strength, and epinephrine and norepinephrine act similarly. If a resistance to blood flow exists in the arteries, the heart responds over time by an enlargement of its muscle mass, known as **cardiac hypertrophy**.

BLOOD PRESSURE

The heart provides the pumping force to build up blood pressure. The elastic arterial system helps sustain that pressure between heartbeats. However, another important element is the peripheral resistance. This is the resistance to flow provided by the *diameter* of the small *arteries* and *arterioles*. Blood pressure is a function of both cardiac output and peripheral resistance.

Blood pressure is described in terms of the **systolic pressure**, the arterial pressure reached as a result of the heart's beat and the **diastolic pressure**, the point to which the pressure falls before it is reinforced by another beat.

In dogs, the mean blood pressure (determined from the systolic and diastolic values) is about 100 mm Hg in the aorta of the dog. The mean pressure falls as blood travels through the vascular system, affected by resistance, and when the systemic arterioles are finally reached, there is little or no pulse.

Venous return is vital to ventricular filling and cardiac output. Its return is accomplished by the **muscle pump** and **respiratory pump**; both are dependent upon the presence of the one-way valves in veins. Whenever local muscle contraction presses on veins, venous blood is forced toward the heart because of these venous valves. During exercise, the action of venous valves can result in a substantial movement of venous blood. Whenever the chest

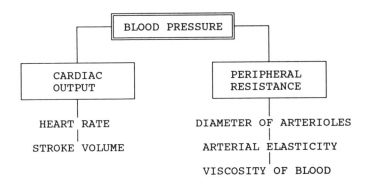

Factors in Blood Pressure This diagram illustrates important factors affecting blood pressure. Influences on cardiac output and peripheral resistance are also listed.

expands by movement of the rib cage and contraction of the muscular diaphragm between the abdomen and thorax (chest), pressure in the chest is lowered and blood easily flows into the chest area; this is quite important during exercise.

An adequate **blood volume** is essential to a normal blood pressure. The elastic arterial system must be appropriately filled, and the venous system must contain a suitable volume in order to assure good venous return.

Fluid intake and retention affect blood volume. **Hemorrhage** results in a loss of water (blood), and **edema** indicates the loss of water from the blood into the interstitial compartment. Under normal conditions, the kidney plays a major role in maintaining the composition and volume of the blood; it does so through the functions of the **antidiuretic hormone** (ADH) and the hormone **aldosterone**, which are discussed in the chapters The Endocrine System and The Urinary System.

Other factors affect your dog's level of hydration and, thereby, blood volume. Cells sensitive to osmotic force, especially the sodium concentration (**osmoreceptors**), are located in the **hypothalamus**. They function with the hormone ADH to regulate water conservation or loss by the kidney.

Other blood-transported (**humoral**) substances that affect blood pressure include **histamine**, a powerful vasodilator; **prostaglandins**, some vasoconstrictors, others vasodilators; **carbon dioxide**, a vasodilator; **lactic acid** and other metabolic acids as vasodilators. A temperature increase brings about vasodilation by both local and reflex action.

Blood pressure is affected by the blood's **viscosity**, which is related to its ability to flow, an effect similar to peripheral resistance. In **anemia**, blood is less viscous because fewer red blood cells are present. Plasma protein concentration also can be quite significant in affecting viscosity. The plasma proteins determine the volume of water that remains inside the vascular system because they are osmotically active across the capillary wall (see below).

THE CAPILLARY AND THE HEALTH OF CELLS

As often mentioned, each body cell lives in the rather optimal and constant environment provided by the blood. The extensive network of microscopic blood capillaries is required to support this environment.

The thin capillary wall freely allows water and **electrolytes** to pass through it, but is relatively impermeable to plasma proteins. Therefore, blood proteins exert a small, but critical, osmotic force that helps hold fluid inside the vessels. The opposing force, the blood pressure in the capillary, tends to force fluid out of the capillary as a **protein-free filtrate**.

When fluid accumulates in the tissue spaces, the condition is called edema. Some possible causes are: (1) a high capillary pressure from dilation of arterioles; (2) high capillary pressure brought about by pressure on veins, e.g., blood clots in veins, tourniquet action by an unattended leash; (3) a low plasma protein

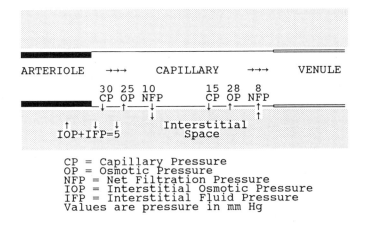

```
ARTERIOLE    →→→      CAPILLARY       →→→     VENULE

         30 25 10              15 28  8
         CP OP NFP             CP OP NFP
         ↓—↑—↓                 ↓—↑—↑
              ↓                        ↑
       ↑    ↓   ↓        Interstitial
       IOP+IFP=5            Space
```

CP = Capillary Pressure
OP = Osmotic Pressure
NFP = Net Filtration Pressure
IOP = Interstitial Osmotic Pressure
IFP = Interstitial Fluid Pressure
Values are pressure in mm Hg

Fluid and Osmotic Forces in Capillaries   The dynamic movement of water and solutes between blood and tissue fluid is illustrated for a typical capillary. The capillary pressure (CP) is the blood pressure remaining at this vascular level. Capillary fluid exchange is influenced by the osmotic pressure (OP), caused by large plasma protein molecules that cannot pass through the capillary wall, and the tissue (interstitial) fluid osmotic pressure (IOP). At any point along the capillary, the net filtration pressure (NFP) is a result of the interactions of all these forces. In contrast to ordinary tissue capillaries, lung capillaries have low pressure and usually do not filter, while renal capillaries have high pressure and filter easily.

concentration; and (4) damaged capillary walls (e.g., from certain toxins) that leak and reduce their effectiveness as osmotic agents.

Some **diuretic** medications reduce the kidney's reabsorption of sodium. This results in increased urine volume; the loss of body fluid may reduce the edema. However, the primary cause of edema must be identified by your veterinarian and corrected.

THE LYMPHATIC SYSTEM

The **lymphatic system** begins as capillarylike structures and drains the interstitial spaces. Areas in their walls function as valves so that fluid (**lymph**) and material can enter.

The lymphatic channels lead through **lymph nodes**, which are populated with cells of the immune system. This association with the immune system permits infectious organisms and other particles to be filtered out at the nodes and be rendered less threatening to the body. Lymph ducts have internal one-way valves and the movement of lymph along its ducts results from body movements. Lymph fluid returns to the blood at veins near the heart. As might be expected, lymphatic vessels assist in reducing edema, but edema may result from blockage of this system when certain parasites infect and damage lymph nodes.

EXERCISE

Although exercise for your dog is closely related to cardiovascular fitness and function, many other physiological considerations must be brought to the study of exercise.

The loss of muscle mass and the increase of fat tissue that characterize aging impair activity. The muscles of older animals have less red pigment, **myoglobin**, which is able to store small amounts of oxygen. Activity becomes limited because compounds that are the immediate source of energy for muscle metabolism and contraction are less abundant. These are **adenosine triphosphate** (ATP) and related **creatine phosphate** (CP). Similarly, all enzyme activities that use oxygen seem restricted.

Finally, connective tissue changes in older dogs result in less joint freedom and slower relaxation of muscles following a contraction. These factors limit the capacity for bursts of activity.

When older dogs begin moderate exercise, it takes longer for their circulation to reach a functional capacity that supplies their oxygen needs. Attention to "warm-up" activities is important, especially for older dogs. Clearly, the circulation of blood is important in sustaining physical activity.

The average maximum heart rate is lower in older dogs for a number of reasons. Cardiac output, a function of heart rate and stroke volume, is also reduced in the aged. Filling is hampered by a loss of elasticity of the cardiac muscle because of connective tissue changes in it. Some cardiac enlargement is common and this may help keep the stroke output almost unchanged.

Electrocardiograms (ECGs) reveal some of the changes in heart function that affect exercise. A veterinarian may be able to recognize ECG changes that indicate insufficient oxygen metabolism in heart muscle. Ventricular **extrasystoles** (extra beats of the ventricles) may be brought on by exercise. Abnormal exercise electrocardiograms increase in frequency with age.

In addition to the above factors, adequacy of venous return, pulmonary efficiency, general hydration and blood volume, and blood pressure are more likely to be compromised in the elderly. Oxygen transport is dependent on pulmonary ventilation and blood flow; blood hemoglobin levels and oxygen-carrying capacity; and systemic blood flow as it is affected by cardiac output, blood pressure, and peripheral resistance.

Anemia is common in the aged and may have several causes. Even when there is good oxygen delivery, older animals may be less able to extract it from the blood. A reduction in some tissue enzymes involved in the process is a likely factor. Also, general vascular regulatory mechanisms may not direct the blood flow to the active muscle as efficiently as in young individuals. A fat older dog may divert a great proportion of blood flow to the mechanisms used for heat loss.

The limitations to prolonged activity also involve the ability to regulate body temperature, the maintenance of body fluid and electrolytes, and the availability of energy-producing substances such as fat, glucose, and glycogen. The thermal insulation from fat and impaired circulation can result in a dangerous rise in temperature. This is more common in the elderly.

Large fluid losses are less well accommodated by older dogs whose kidney function and water intake may not have maintained adequate water and electrolyte reserves. Severe exercise in the elderly may actually provoke kidney failure in those with renal disease.

A widely held hope is that a physically active life-style throughout life will contribute to longevity. Until recently, that did not seem to be supported with evidence. Most data support the conclusion that both sedentary and active animals lose oxygen intake ability at similar rates. However, regularly active dogs start with and should maintain a superior capacity over sedentary ones.

Also, the genetic effects of selecting breed characteristics may have intentionally or unintentionally selected athletic features in dogs. For example, Greyhounds and similar dogs have quite large hearts compared with other breeds.

The conclusion is that *regular exercise benefits all ages by enhancing the dog's ability for physical activities*. However, the physiological advantages of exercise do not seem to persist after an exercise program ceases to be a part of an animal's life-style. Aerobic capacity diminishes with age at about the same rate in active and nonactive humans. Exercise continued throughout life does not seem to confer more than a small extension of life span. Yet, many other benefits of exercise exist and should provide sufficient reason to keep dogs reasonably active.

THE AGING CARDIOVASCULAR SYSTEM

HEART AND BLOOD VESSELS

During aging, the ventricular size often increases (**ventricular hypertrophy**), but this may be caused by disease rather than age alone. Many hearts become covered over by a layer of fat, and considerable fat is associated with the membranous sac around the heart (**pericardium**). This deposition of fat probably reflects disease, not normal, healthy aging.

Cardiac output decreases about 30 percent by the last one-third of a dog's normal life span. Degenerative changes in heart valves and heart muscle are evident in older dogs.

With age, heart valves become thicker and more rigid. This predisposes older dogs to failing heart function. Blood is able to flow backward through incompetent valves, decreasing the heart's efficiency. Also, these valves accumulate lipids and develop calcium deposits. The bases of the valvular cusps may form **adhesions**.

The resting heart rate decreases throughout life, as does the maximum rate. Elderly dogs commonly have much less performance reserve because of cardiac disease. These are some myocardial changes that are more universal.

CARDIOVASCULAR DISEASES

Diseases of the Heart Valves

The functional impairment of heart valves, **chronic valvular heart disease**, is a very common cause of heart failure in the dog. It occurs more commonly in males, and small breeds seem more susceptible. When the A-V valve (between the left atrium and left ventricle—**mitral valve**) is incompetent, pressure will back up in the lungs, causing pulmonary edema. If the left atrium becomes engorged with enough blood, it may cause pressure on lung airways.

Dogs with chronic valvular heart disease have heart murmurs that can be heard through the veterinarian's stethoscope. These murmurs are usually from noises made by blood being forced backward past leaky valves, often through the valves that separate the left atrium and left ventricle. The heart must work harder whenever any of the heart valves are impaired. Exercise intolerance and, in severe cases, fainting (**syncope**) may be primary signs of heart valve leakage. Coughing and weight loss may be secondarily caused symptoms. However, many dogs with heart murmur show no other signs of heart disease.

HEART FAILURE

Unlike humans, aging dogs rarely have coronary heart disease caused by fatty plaque deposits (**atherosclerosis**), and hardening of the arteries (**arteriosclerosis**) is uncommon. However, it is usually failure of heart valves, leading to overburdening the heart muscle or deterioration of the heart muscle itself (**cardiomyopathy**), that leads to heart failure in the dog. Flawed heart valve action may excessively burden the heart and result in lower blood pressure and inadequate coronary flow. Compensatory heart enlargement may occur.

Veterinarians may classify heart failure as **left heart failure** or **right heart failure**, depending on effects on other parts of the body. When the left ventricle is inadequate, pulmonary edema results. This is generally what is meant by **congestive heart failure**. If the right ventricle is unable to empty effectively, pressure goes up in the veins and capillaries of the body. This causes swelling in tissues and fluid accumulation in the abdomen (**ascites**). Right heart failure commonly occurs following failure of the left ventricle.

Congestive Heart Failure

Whenever the heart chronically fails to pump the venous blood returned to it, there is a rise in the venous pressure. This rise acts to increase the pressure all the way back to the capillaries as a tourniquet would. Failure of the left ventricle is especially dangerous because its venous supply is from the lungs. High pressure in the pulmonary vein causes congestion in the lungs, fluid in the air spaces (**alveoli**), and failure of effective pulmonary gas exchange.

As congestive heart failure gets worse, exercise intolerance increases, weight loss occurs in the face of apparently good appetite, coughing increases, and, finally, fainting spells may occur. The ''air hunger'' experienced by an affected dog is extremely distressful, and the ability of the heart to empty must be improved for survival. Because the heart muscle is commonly at fault, even if brought on by faulty valves, the prognosis is not good in many cases, but ways to relieve the burden exist and may improve the quality of life for a time.

Reducing the blood volume by restricting salt intake may be helpful in reducing the edema. If body weight is excessive, it must be reduced. Medical treatments include reducing blood volume with diuretics, reducing resistance to blood flow, and reducing the work of the heart with vasodilators. There has also been success with increasing the strength of the heart with **cardiac glycosides** (e.g., **digitalis**), and aiding respiration with drugs that dilate the bronchi in the lungs. Many of these drugs have serious side effects, and your veterinarian should discuss them with you.

Abnormal Heart Rhythms

When the heartbeat results from the normal, regularly spaced impulses from the S-A node, the impulses spread over the atrial muscle, discharge the A-V node, and travel through the ventricular muscle. This is referred to as **sinus rhythm**. This is the normal rhythm of the heart. Deviations from this rate or pattern are called **arrhythmias**, and while some are relatively benign, others are quite serious.

When the conducting tissue that transmits the cardiac impulse from the atrium to the ventricle fails, a **heart block** is said to exist. It may be a *partial* heart block in which the impulse successfully crosses from the atrium at intervals. For example, a two-to-one heart block means that every other impulse crosses satisfactorily. In a *complete* heart block no impulses cross. In this case, the ventricle may begin its own, but slower, rhythm. When the impulse is initiated at the A-V node instead of the S-A node, the impulse travels through the atria at the same time that it sweeps over the ventricle muscle. This is known as a **nodal rhythm**. **Tachycardia** is the term for a rapid heart rate. **Bradycardia** is used to describe a slow heart rate. The electrocardiogram (ECG) is very helpful in aiding the veterinarian to determine the exact nature of arrhythmias.

Sometimes an impairment of the heart muscle shows in a chaotic pattern of contractions (**fibrillation**). The heart's pumping action is defeated if the ventricle fibrillates, and emergency attention is required. Atrial fibrillation has less immediate consequences, but it must be evaluated by your veterinarian. Fibrillation is caused by an abnormality in the system that initiates and transmits the impulse controlling the heart cycle. The heart may be ''shocked'' by using a **defibrillator**, which actually stops it momentarily and allows a normal heart cycle to return. The same procedure may reinstate the heartbeat after **cardiac arrest** (heart stoppage). Medication may reduce the likelihood of recurrence of fibrillation.

Failure of or erratic behavior of the normal pacemaker function of the S-A node may require implantation of a small electronic unit that supplies regular stimulation to the heart. These stimuli are quite below the level that can be felt consciously. **Cardiac pacemakers** have been used in humans for about two decades. Much early experimental work in developing the device was conducted in dogs, and they are finally being used in veterinary practice. These instruments are considered useful whenever it has been established that the S-A node does not initiate an impulse at the correct frequency. In other cases, a complete or partial heart block may need an artificial impulse to maintain adequate ventricular rate. These heart conduction problems may be associated with Addison's disease (**hypoadrenocorticolism;** see the chapter The Endocrine System), activity of parasympathetic nerves to the heart, high blood potassium levels, kidney failure, or certain other diseases.

Cardiovascular Shock

Blood pressure that falls below the level necessary to supply the brain and coronary vessels constitutes **cardiovascular shock**. Primary causes include failure of the heart to pump, loss of blood volume needed to fill the system, or massive vasodilation (as in **anaphylactic shock** resulting from an immune reaction that releases histamine).

In the elderly dog, some medications needed for other ailments interfere with cardiovascular reflexes. Loss of blood by hemorrhage or loss of body fluid because of kidney malfunctions are serious complications. Protein malnutrition may reduce the blood volume to create an unstable circulatory system. Your veterinarian must establish the cause and correct it if possible. Because cardiovascular shock can be fatal, transfusion of blood or saline solution may be needed as well.

Pericardial Disease

The heart is surrounded by a rather tough membrane, the pericardium. At times, this membrane may become infected (**pericarditis**). The inflammation results in accumulation of bloody fluid in the pericardial space. Also, sterile fluid may collect in the pericardial space as a consequence of congestive heart failure. Occasionally, parasites or tumors in the pericardial area may be responsible for such fluid accumulation. Owners may first notice a swelling of the abdomen (ascites), fatigue, and respiratory distress. The problem is a restriction placed on proper filling of the heart by the pressure around the heart. It has much the same effect as congestive heart failure even if that condition is not present. In this case, the heart cannot adequately fill, rather than empty. The effect still makes venous and capillary pressure rise.

Pericardial fluid accumulation can be diagnosed by changes in heart sounds, electrocardiograms, X-ray images, and echocardiography, which is a means of using sound to get an image of the heart's size and shape. Whenever infection is involved, antibiotics are appropriate. In any case, the fluid may be aspirated by needle, temporarily relieving the heart of the blockage to adequate filling.

Heartworm (Dirofilaria) Infection

The parasitic worm *Dirofilaria immitis* has become common in dogs, especially in regions with high mosquito activity. The organism is transmitted by mosquitoes that have picked up larvae from an infected animal. It is found in other animals and, rarely, in humans. It is not a specific disease of elderly dogs, but time and opportunity for exposure may influence infection rate.

Great numbers of adult worms (**dirofilaria**), four to twelve inches long, may reside in the chambers on the right side of the heart—250 have been reported in a single dog. A female worm can give birth to thousands of **microfilariae** per day. These very small stages of the organism circulate in the dog's blood, but do not mature in the host. They must pass through a secondary host, a mosquito, to start the process that leads to maturity. A number of days after a mosquito's blood meal, the larvae become infective and will become adults in the next dog bitten.

Adult dirofilaria live in the pulmonary artery, right atrium, and right ventricle. These are all areas of low oxygen tension. They can impede blood flow to the lungs by occupying space in the heart and interfering with heart valve closure. Sometimes these worms live in the veins leading to the right atrium, slowing liver blood flow and promoting its failure. Symptoms of liver failure can develop rapidly and cause death quickly.

Medication should never be used that could suddenly kill the worms, allowing their bodies to enter lung circulation. Death may quickly follow a worm embolism in the lung. *Your veterinarian should establish whether worms are already present or not, and then recommend a course of treatment or prevention.*

Weight loss, a characteristic cough, and general weakness are common symptoms of heartworm infection. The severity varies with the number of worms and their specific location. As the condition becomes more advanced, the consequences of congestive heart failure become apparent, and liver failure may follow.

Diagnosis is usually established by finding microfilariae in a blood sample if they are sufficiently numerous. However, if both sexes of worm are not present, microfilariae will not be produced. Adult worms may not yet be sexually mature. It has been proposed that some dogs produce antibodies that keep their blood free of microfilariae. X-ray examination of the heart and repeated blood examination may be required for diagnosis.

Several drugs are available for treatment, but must always be used under careful veterinary supervision. Not only must the adult worms be killed under controlled conditions (e.g., with thiacetarsamide), the microfilariae must be destroyed (e.g., with dithiazanine). These drugs have various side effects independent of worm embolism, further calling for careful attention by your veterinarian. Occasionally, worms are removed surgically.

Once a dog is shown to be free of dirofilaria in any stage, drugs such as diethylcarbamazine will kill infective larvae before they mature. Keeping dogs behind screens and indoors when mosquitoes are active and using some environmental mosquito control can help reduce infection. However, these efforts are not completely effective.

10

The Urinary System: Kidney and Bladder Function and Health

THE ROLES OF THE KIDNEY

Most people think of the kidney as a blood filter, and that is certainly one of its major functions. Filtering the blood separates the fluid and small **solutes** from blood cells and large protein molecules. Further actions produce urine containing waste products. The blood's pH (acid-base balance), solute concentrations, and volume are adjusted to optimum levels. The kidney is also an endocrine organ. It secretes a hormone that controls the production of red blood cells. It has been previously noted that the kidney produces the active form of vitamin D (actually a **steroid hormone**). Also, the kidney produces an enzyme that converts a plasma protein into a powerful vasoconstrictive hormone. The dog's kidney is the specific target of two hormones that influence its handling of water and sodium.

The functional units (**nephrons**) in the kidneys are more abundant than needed in young dogs. A dog's kidneys may still meet the body's needs after loss of up to 80 percent of their nephrons. One kidney can be lost (or be absent at birth) and the remaining one is able to serve the body quite well. However, with age or certain diseases, this reserve may be so diminished that there are serious consequences.

Kidney diseases are important, but not universal, features of aging. The

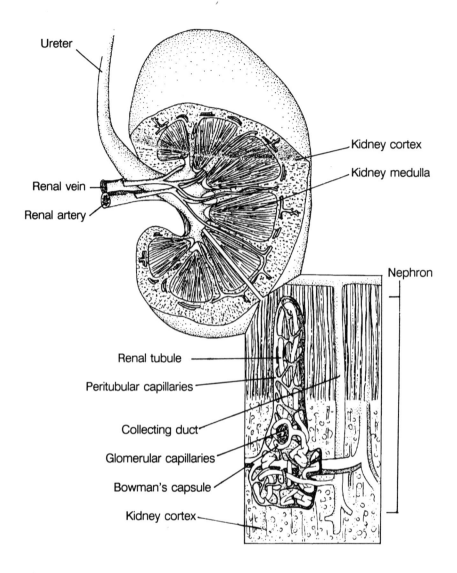

The Mammalian Kidney The kidneys, supplied with blood at high pressure, are designed for filtering and modifying a great amount of blood. The outer renal cortex contains a rich supply of capillaries in which a cell-free filtrate of the blood is formed. The inner medulla portion contains tubules, capillaries, and collecting ducts that modify the filtrate and deliver it to the ureters. The inset is a diagram of a functional unit, a nephron.

110

average age for beginning kidney failure in dogs is about seven years. It is claimed to be the second most common cause of nonaccidental death in dogs. Older dogs' kidneys have limited ability to compensate for challenges brought on by other diseases.

The dog's two kidneys (**renal organs**) are located in the abdomen near the vertebral column. The connection between the kidneys and the **aorta** (large central artery) is short.

THE BLADDER

The **urinary bladder** is located in the lower (**pelvic**) area of the abdomen. It receives urine from the kidneys by way of two muscular-walled **ureters**. The bladder empties to the outside of the body through the single tubular **urethra**.

No alteration of urine takes place in the bladder. It is only a storage vessel. Smooth muscle fibers of the ureter walls produce peristaltic waves of contraction that propel urine toward the bladder. Two muscle rings (**sphincters**) can prevent urine from leaving the bladder and entering the urethra. The **internal urethral sphincter** in the neck of the bladder is pulled forward by contraction of the bladder and opened. The **external urethral sphincter** surrounds the upper part of the urethra. It must relax for urination to occur.

The smooth muscle walls of the urinary bladder in a healthy dog maintain relatively constant pressure on its contents to some limit, regardless of its volume. When the volume exceeds this limit, pressure increases and a conscious desire to urinate develops. Central nervous system activity can inhibit the nervous reflexes and, therefore, delay bladder emptying. This is the basis for a dog's ability to become "housebroken."

The act of urination occurs when a spinal-level reflex contracts the bladder muscles, elevates the internal urethral sphincter, and inhibits the external urethral sphincter. Dogs with certain spinal injuries lose the ability to control the bladder sphincter. They become **incontinent**.

BLOOD VESSEL (VASCULAR) FEATURES

Blood filtration by the kidney requires a substantial volume of blood flow at relatively high pressure. To accomplish this, the nephrons have a unique blood supply. The arteries leading to each kidney are short and derived from the large aorta. Thus, blood arriving at the kidney loses little pressure since leaving the heart. In the cortex of the kidney, complex capillary beds are intimately associated with each nephron tubule.

As the fluid filtered from blood travels through nephron tubules, the filtrate composition is modified in three ways. A few substances are actively secreted into the tubular lumen. These substances are added to those already in the filtrate. Drugs and other substances that are secreted include penicillin, morphine, and aspirin. Hydrogen ions are secreted, providing one means of protecting the body from excess acid accumulation. The body's metabolic products **uric acid**, **prostaglandins**, **fatty acids**, **epinephrine**, **dopamine**, **histamine**, and **bile salts** are known to be secreted. The substance **para-aminohippuric acid (PAH)** is so effectively secreted, in addition to being filtered, that measurement of the removal of PAH from blood passing through the kidney can be used to measure the **effective renal blood flow**.

A second means of modifying the tubular filtrate is **reabsorption**. This is the main process of modifying the filtrate. Reabsorption resembles secretion, although the direction is from the lumen back into the peritubular capillary blood. Ordinarily, filtered glucose is completely transported back. Sodium is filtered freely and is mostly reabsorbed. Amino acids, lactate ions, Cl^-, HCO_3^-, and K^+ are others.

The third way in which tubular filtrate is modified is by substances returning to the blood across the tubular wall by **diffusion**. The movement of water is the most important example of diffusion. An enormous amount of water is returned from the filtrate, primarily because of the active removal of sodium from the filtrate. As sodium is removed, the water left behind is "purer." The water itself has become more concentrated (i.e., "pure") relative to blood, so it diffuses down its concentration gradient toward the blood; in other words, it follows the sodium. Also, as sodium and water return to the blood, other substances are left behind and become more concentrated as the water leaves. Then, these substances diffuse from areas of high concentration (the tubule) to areas of lower concentration (the blood).

As previously mentioned, PAH can be used to measure the effective renal blood flow. The **polysaccharide inulin** (*not* insulin) is known to be freely filtered, but inulin is neither secreted nor reabsorbed. This makes it useful to measure the **glomerular filtration rate** (GFR) because filtration alone accounts for its presence in the urine. Just as PAH can be said to be "cleared" from blood in passage, the same **clearance** concept can be applied to substances such as inulin.

Knowledge of the GFR is of considerable importance in evaluating the health of the kidney. Loss of glomeruli because of disease, failure to function because of low blood pressure following hemorrhage or weak heart function, or the congenital absence of kidney tissue lowers the GFR. Renal blood flow and GFR are reduced during periods of strong emotion, pain, and vigorous exercise. These are circumstances when blood flow is diverted to other areas of the body.

Glucose is conserved by active transport reabsorption. However, if the blood sugar (glucose) is above normal, the reabsorptive system may be unable to accommodate the larger amounts in the filtrate. The kidney is not at fault in **diabetes mellitus**; high plasma glucose filtered in excessive amounts accounts for incomplete glucose reabsorption.

The kidneys and the lungs of your dog are vital to the regulation of the narrow range of blood pH required by the body. The lungs provide a quick means of modifying the acid-base condition of the blood. Lungs retain or excrete CO_2, which is largely transported as carbonic acid (H_2CO_3) or bicarbonate (HCO_3^-). On the other hand, the kidney is slower in correcting pH changes, but such changes are more substantial and stable. The pH of the body fluids is carefully maintained in health and adjusted whenever metabolism, vomiting, diarrhea, or respiratory impairment tends to shift the acid-base balance.

CONTROL OF KIDNEY FUNCTION

One endocrine control system for kidney function may be illustrated by its relationship to the disease **diabetes insipidus** (''tasteless'' diabetes), which is unrelated to diabetes mellitus. It certainly involves the kidney's function, but not necessarily a diseased kidney. It is characterized by a dilute urine that is produced in much greater volume than normal.

A basis for the disease is the failure of the **hypothalamus** to produce adequate **antidiuretic hormone** (ADH), which is released from the **posterior**

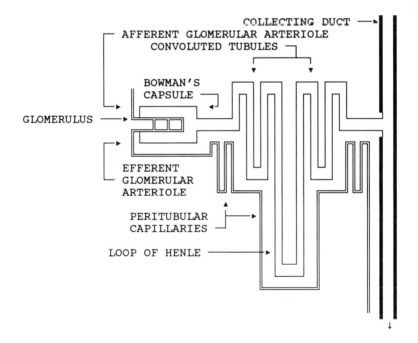

The Nephron This is a diagram of the kidney's primary functioning unit, the nephron. An afferent glomerular arteriole drains into the capillaries of the glomerulus, then into the efferent glomerular arteriole, and finally into the capillary bed that surrounds the rest of the nephron. Filtrate from capillaries is collected by Bowman's capsule and flows through the proximal convoluted tubule, the loop of Henle, and the distal convoluted tubule. During this passage, the filtrate is converted into urine by secretion, reabsorption, and diffusion processes. A collecting duct collects urine from a number of nephrons and delivers the urine, via the ureter, to the urinary bladder.

pituitary gland (see the chapter The Endocrine System). This hormone acts on the nephron and the collecting ducts to increase the permeability to water so that it can follow the sodium that is reabsorbed. Thus, lack of ADH causes excess water to be excreted—a **diuresis.**

Another hormone, the adrenocortical steroid **aldosterone** (see the chapter The Endocrine System), helps control kidney (renal) function. It aids in handling sodium and water. The endocrine-based condition known as **Addison's disease** is characterized by a failure of the adrenal cortex to produce an appropriate amount of aldosterone. In this condition, severe dehydration resulting from sodium loss may prove fatal.

ADH, aldosterone, and parathyroid hormone have long been recognized for their effects on renal function. Currently, over twenty hormones and physiological mediators appear involved in some way, to some extent, in kidney activity. Some are steroids such as glucocorticoids, progesterone, and vitamin D. Peptide hormones that have been studied include **glucagon**, insulin, **angiotensin II, calcitonin, atrial natriuretic factor**, and **thyroid hormones**.

The Kidney as an Endocrine Gland

The kidney's role in production of active vitamin D has been mentioned (see the chapter The Endocrine System). Another substance produced by the kidney is a hormone (or growth factor), **erythropoietin**, that acts on the **bone marrow** to cause red blood cell production.

AGING AND THE URINARY SYSTEM

ANATOMICAL AND PHYSIOLOGICAL CHANGES

The kidney reaches maximum size in early adulthood. Thereafter, the weight and volume decrease throughout life. A greater decrease is seen in the cortex, which contains mainly nephrons and capillaries. Microscopic examination shows deformed capillaries through which blood no longer flows. These changes seem to be fundamental to aging, and help explain the reduced GFR and renal blood flow seen in aging. However, old dogs are known to be prone to kidney disease. Both the ability to concentrate the urine and to produce dilute urine is reduced in the aged.

When disease of the kidney or other tissue challenges the elderly dog, the lowered reserve of renal function becomes serious because its overall homeostatic role is vital. Events such as diarrhea and vomiting may be life-threatening to an older dog because of subsequent salt/water and pH imbalances that depend upon the kidney for correction.

When one kidney is removed, it is characteristic for the other one to undergo compensatory hypertrophy (grow larger) with an important increase in functional capacity. The older an animal is, the less compensatory hypertrophy occurs—and the retained kidney already will have had the reduced function concomitant with age. Thus, the loss of a kidney in an old dog is quite serious.

The urinary bladder, ureters, and urethra are structures that depend on the proper function of nerves and muscles. Loss of muscle tone results in difficulty in emptying the bladder or, in other cases, **incontinence** because sphincters function inadequately. The bladder capacity for urine volume also appears to diminish with age.

DISEASES OF THE URINARY SYSTEM

Kidney and Bladder Stones (Uroliths)

The formation of kidney and bladder stones (**urolithiasis**) is sometimes "silent," but it is a serious condition. It may be a painful condition when the stone attempts to pass through the ureter or urethra. The stones may be in the form of sandlike granules or as large masses. Unlike humans, dogs have bladder stones much more frequently than kidney stones.

A primary reason for stone formation is oversaturation of dissolved material because of the kidney's water reabsorption. When high concentrations are reached, crystals or amorphous masses precipitate. Changes in urine pH may influence this process because some substances are more soluble in either acid or alkaline environments. Atypical diets that constantly promote a urine with a pH at either extreme may initiate stone formation. It is obvious that inadequate water intake or excessive loss produces a water-conserving reabsorption that markedly concentrates the urine. Kidney infections may encourage kidney stone formation by releasing precipitated protein masses and cellular material into the urine to serve as a place for the stones to form.

Breeds that have been mentioned as being predisposed to **uroliths** are Pekingese, Dachshunds, and Cocker Spaniels. Dalmatians commonly have uroliths, but their situation has special features.

Dalmatians, while susceptible to various uroliths (nearly one-fourth of their uroliths are phosphates), warrant attention because they are a breed that makes and excretes **uric acid**, as do humans and the great apes. Thus, they often form uroliths composed of **urates** (salts of uric acid). This condition relates to the Dalmatian's inability to convert uric acid to **allantoin**, which would be more easily handled. Individuals of this breed may have a recessive genetic defect affecting their liver's metabolism of uric acid. Urate uroliths may occur in other breeds, especially if liver disease alters their metabolism of uric acid.

In the past, abdominal surgery was the only way to remove a kidney stone. Today, research seeks to find safe substances that will dissolve uroliths. Conventional surgery is giving way to sonic fracturing (**lithotripsy**) of stones by focusing special sound waves on them. Another technique uses a probe that administers shock waves and is placed in the pelvis of the kidney or elsewhere.

With this method, the particles of the stone are rinsed out. This method has been more successful in humans because of their size and other anatomical features.

Cytocentesis is the term used for a procedure in which a needle is inserted into the bladder through the abdominal wall, often under local anesthesia. Sometimes a veterinarian may be able to feel relatively small uroliths and, by massage, cause them to be mobilized and passed. In other cases, uroliths may be rinsed out of the urethra by expert use of catheters passed through the urethra. Sometimes, with knowledge of the chemical composition of a stone, a rinsing solution may be chosen that will dissolve the stone.

If blockage in the kidney, ureter, or urethra is removed, there is a good chance function will return. However, stretching the bladder and injury to its sphincters or nerve supply may have lingering consequences. Of course, *reasonable dietary practices and adequate water intake as a regular life-style pattern can help prevent formation of uroliths, even for those that may have inherited a predisposition for them.*

Infections of the Urinary System

The urethra, the bladder, the ureter, and the kidney are subject to infection more frequently in the elderly than in the young. **Cystitis** is infection of the urinary bladder without regard to the organism responsible. Often the offending organisms are common ones that are found on the surfaces of the body or in the anal area. The symptoms of cystitis include abdominal pain, frequent and strong urges to urinate, burning pain in the urethra upon urination, and sometimes **hematuria** (blood in the urine).

Females experience cystitis much more frequently, probably because their urethras are much shorter than males'. It is essential that good medical treatment be given because some infections lead to more serious conditions, even chronic renal infections that are resistant to treatment. In addition to antibiotics, treatments designed to change the pH of the urine may help make the bladder more inhospitable to an offending organism. Drinking fluids freely may be desirable. The limited capacity of the elderly dog to adjust salt/water balance must be kept in mind in order to avoid a serious condition called *water toxicity.* Clearly, competent veterinary care is indicated for old dogs with kidney infection, not home remedies.

Pyelonephritis (or **nephritis**) means infection of the whole kidney with one or more types of bacteria—a life-threatening infection. **Glomerulonephritis** refers to nephritis that particularly involves the glomerular capillaries. Kidney infection may be **acute** or **chronic** and symptoms may be slight to severe. When allowed to continue, nephritis leads to renal failure and **uremia**, a condition in which waste products (urea, **creatinine**, uric acid, etc.), ordinarily excreted, accumulate in the blood. The uremic condition may first be noticed by symptoms such as abdominal pain, chills and fever, nausea, vomiting, diarrhea, and lethargy.

Prostatitis (inflammation of the **prostate gland**) occurs in older dogs (see the chapter The Reproductive System). In this condition, cyst formation is common, and infection of them leads to abscesses that are difficult to treat. As in age-related prostatic enlargement, castration is often carried out to remove the growth stimulus of **testosterone**.

Chronic Renal Failure

Chronic renal failure, which usually occurs in older dogs, is caused by loss of functional kidney tissue. This differs from **acute renal failure**, which is usually associated with factors outside the kidneys. As the condition becomes more severe, uremia develops. Treatment is as complex as the many factors that can be involved in chronic renal failure. Of course, diagnosis and treatment of the causes of a related disease are imperative. Because of the adverse effects on total body function, management of the symptoms must be the first order, because death may intervene before causes can be found and corrected.

Acute Renal Failure

Uremia also results from **acute renal failure**, which is a relatively sudden failure of the kidney to perform normally, including inability to produce a normal urine volume. Failure because of renal causes occurs in individuals of any age. Especially in the elderly dog, considerable loss of body fluids and electrolytes caused by vomiting or diarrhea may exceed the renal reserve. An inadequate intake of fluids, complicated by the use of diuretics, may also exceed the kidney's tolerance.

Acute renal failure may follow the stress of surgery or heart trouble. Urinary tract obstruction can also damage the kidney by retention of urine in the kidney pelvis under pressure. Another condition of this sort is the obstruction of the urethra by an enlarged prostate gland (see the chapter The Reproductive System). The kidney is sometimes damaged by drug-induced immunological reactions, drug toxicity (e.g., certain antibiotics), **bacteremias** (generalized, blood-borne bacterial infections), and obstruction of renal blood vessels. *Treatment is directed toward prompt reestablishment of water/electrolyte balance and specific treatment of the primary assault on the kidney.*

Incontinence and Frequent Urination

Urinary incontinence (failure to delay or control urination) occurs primarily in middle-aged to elderly dogs. Urinary bladder and other urinary tract infections are the most common causes, although nervous system dysfunction is sometimes to blame. Bladder tumors may limit the capacity of the bladder to hold urine. These tumors seem to appear most commonly around nine years of age.

Passing of urine is a spinal reflex that is subject to control by the central nervous system; somatic motor and autonomic nerves supply innervation to the walls and sphincters of the bladder. Incontinence is more common in old dogs, especially spayed bitches. Treatment with estrogen may be helpful for them. Loss of control may be total, occur intermittently, or only at times when high intra-abdominal pressure is experienced, as when coughing or barking.

Enlargement of the prostate gland is present in many male dogs over five years of age. This appears to cause less difficulty in dogs than in humans, in whom it is known as **benign prostatic hyperplasia** (BPH). In older dogs, an enlarged prostate, which is usually noncancerous, may produce enough pressure on the urethra or bladder to affect urination. However, the dog's enlarged prostate gland more commonly encroaches upon the rectal area, causing problems with defecation. Treatment of the condition usually includes castration to remove the source of testosterone, as in the case of prostatitis, which supports continued enlargement. The prostate gland is part of the reproductive system and will be further described in the chapter The Reproductive System.

Urinary Tract Tumors and Cancer

Tumors of the kidneys are not common in dogs. But, as with tumors elsewhere in the body, older dogs are favored.

Even malignant and benign tumors of the ureters, bladder and urethra are uncommon. Exceptions are **nephroblastomas**, tumors arising from embryonic tissue and observed in dogs under one year of age. When cancer is present, bloody urine is often the first sign that attracts attention. Discomfort will accompany the obstruction to urine flow caused by the growth of a tumor mass.

Cancer of the prostate in males may be more common. It is mostly seen in dogs over ten years of age. Prostate cancer causes some of the same symptoms seen in benign prostatic enlargement and cystitis—blood in the urine and painful voiding. A veterinarian's skill and knowledge are absolutely necessary to deal with this condition.

11

The Respiratory System

IT IS NOT generally realized that the lungs (**pulmonary system**) are an animal's most extensive and intimate contact with its outside environment. The wide range in the body sizes of dogs makes an illustration difficult. Over 3,000 gallons of air move into and out of the human lungs daily in the resting condition. The amount may be several times greater during high levels of activity. Most of this air reaches the smallest areas of the respiratory system (the **alveoli**), allowing close contact with the blood in the lung capillaries of humans and dogs.

The **pulmonary blood flow** is especially great (see the chapter The Cardiovascular System). *The same amount of blood is pumped through the lungs each minute as is sent through the rest of the body in the same period of time.*

The evolution of the respiratory system freed animals from the sea. However, it did more than that; it allowed animals to develop high metabolic rates that depend on their greater use of oxygen, which is fifty times more abundant on land than in a water environment.

The dog's lungs have developed important barrier and immune functions to protect the rest of the body (see the chapter The Protective Role of the Immune System). The great amount of oxygen subjects lung tissue to the adverse effects of many oxidizing reactions. Certain lung cells play endocrine roles independent of respiration, and many special lung enzymes exist.

To a significantly greater degree than in humans, dogs use their respiratory systems to effect body cooling. The specific mechanism will be described in detail. Understanding it may be life-saving, because dogs are acutely susceptible to confinement in hot, humid environments.

Because there is no significant storage of oxygen, respiratory exchange of oxygen and carbon dioxide must be continuous. Some deterioration is age-related, but many lung diseases are associated with injury because of environmental factors.

In humans in the United States and many other countries, cigarette smoking is the cardinal agent for lung injury; recent information confirms smoking's deleterious secondhand effects on nonsmoking humans, and dogs may be similarly affected. Some pulmonary malfunctions result when other systems fail. In **congestive heart failure**, the inability of the left ventricle of the heart to empty causes congestion in the blood vessels of the lung. The resulting **pulmonary edema** is a major medical emergency (see the chapter The Cardiovascular System).

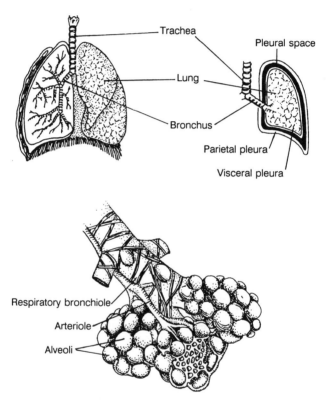

Anatomy of the Lungs   The pulmonary system begins at the mouth and nasal cavities and continues into an area used for breathing and swallowing (nasopharyngeal). Starting at the larynx (voice box), the trachea and branching bronchi, held open by cartilage rings, carry air to the depths of the lungs via the bronchioles. Bronchioles terminate at the alveoli (air sacs), which are surrounded by a rich blood supply. The lungs are surrounded by two pleural membranes. The parietal pleura is attached to the inner chest wall; the visceral pleura covers the outer lung surface. Between the pleurae, a thin layer of lubricant allows easy movements during breathing.

RESPIRATORY ANATOMY AND PHYSIOLOGY

Anatomy and Functional Properties

The air passages begin with the **nasal** (nose) and **oral** (mouth) cavities. The **pharynx** (the common space entering the throat) divides into the **esophagus**, which carries foodstuff into the stomach, and the **trachea**, which leads to the lungs. A flaplike structure, the **epiglottis**, closes the top of the trachea so that food and water enter only the esophagus.

During its travel through the nasal cavity and the pharynx, cold air is warmed and humidified. Evaporation in nasal areas is especially important in the dog's mechanism for body cooling. Air is then moved through the single trachea, the branches called **bronchi**, and the many **bronchiole** branches. Bronchioles give rise to **respiratory bronchioles**, which end in **alveolar ducts** and associated clusters of **alveoli**. Only when air reaches the alveoli is it exposed to **capillaries** of the vascular system. Here, gas exchange can take place.

A dog, depending on its size, may have millions of alveoli, each having a diameter of less than a third of a millimeter. A cluster of alveoli, somewhat resembling a cluster of grapes, is served by a single alveolar duct. An extensive distribution of blood capillaries surround the alveoli. The gases carbon dioxide and oxygen have but two layers of cells to pass through—the capillary wall and the alveolar wall.

The lungs, which have a relatively small blood volume, receive a proportion of the **cardiac output** equal to that sent to the rest of the body. The lungs are organized into lobes on each side of the **thoracic** (chest) cavity. The outer surfaces of the lungs are covered with a membrane called the **visceral pleura**, and the inner surface of the thoracic cavity is similarly covered by the **parietal pleura**. Between the two membranes is a fluid with high lubricating properties. This allows almost friction-free movement and changes in shape during respiratory activity. Painful infection and inflammation of the pleural membranes is referred to as **pleuritis** (**pleurisy**).

The mechanics of breathing increase and decrease the thoracic space. The muscles attached to the ribs (the **intercostal muscles**) reposition the ribs by moving them outward and forward. The **diaphragm**, which separates the thoracic cavity from the abdominal space, contracts and draws it toward the abdomen. Both of these muscular actions increase the space within the thorax. The contraction of other muscles may assist the expulsion of air by forcefully reducing chest capacity.

At rest, however, the return of the thorax to its previous state occurs by the relaxation of the muscles. This occurs because the lungs are quite elastic. In fact, even in the resting position, the lungs exert a significant elastic pull against the chest walls.

About one-third of lung elasticity appears to be from **elastin** and **collagen** fibers. In order to allow the lungs to expand and fill with air with reasonable effort, the moist surfaces of the alveoli are coated with surface-acting agents (**surfactants**) that are produced by lung tissue. Premature puppies may be born before their ability to produce surfactants has been established. They suffer a life-threatening inability to effectively inflate their lungs. Diseases of the lungs in older dogs sometimes involve problems in maintaining surface tension properties.

Lung Volumes

The air in the lungs may be classified in terms of various volumes or the "spaces" they occupy. These are measured with a **spirometer**, an instrument in which air can be captured and its volume measured. The spirometer cannot measure all of the gas in an animal's lungs because all of it cannot be exhaled into the instrument. No matter what, some air remains in the lungs. This amount of remaining air is called the **residual volume**. It is always there and even the most vigorous ventilatory activity must always mix inhaled air with that residual volume.

The amount of air that can be exhaled following a maximum inhalation is known as the **vital capacity**. The vital capacity plus the residual volume is the **total lung capacity**. However, normal breathing at rest represents the movement of much less air. This is a level of respiration that can be extended by either greater inhalation or greater exhalation.

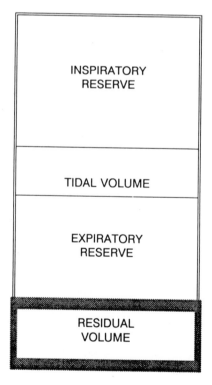

Lung Volume Compartments The tidal volume is the amount of air normally breathed in and out. A greater inspiratory effort will take in the inspiratory volume; maximal expiratory effort will expel the expiratory reserve. The residual volume is always present, and any air breathed in must be mixed with it. The rate of respiration and the size of the tidal and residual volumes determine the composition of the air in the alveoli.

INSPIRATORY RESERVE

TIDAL VOLUME

EXPIRATORY RESERVE

RESIDUAL VOLUME

The amount of air that is turned over with each breath is the **tidal volume**, usually a relatively small volume while a dog is at rest. At the end of a normal exhalation, further effort can usually expel some more—the **expiratory reserve**. Similarly, at the end of a normal resting inspiration, additional air can be inhaled; this is the **inspiratory reserve**.

CONTROL OF RESPIRATION

The central nervous system areas involved in respiration are located in the **pons** and **medulla oblongata** (see the chapter The Central Nervous System). A **pneumotaxic center** (*pneumo-* refers to the lung or respiration) is found in the pons, and its role appears to help make breathing a smoothly coordinated activity. An **apneustic center** (*-pnea* refers to breathing; *apneustic* indicates a cessation of inspiratory activity) is also in the pons.

The apneustic center is activated when the lungs are stretched by *inhalation*. As a result, it "turns off" inhalation and allows *exhalation* to occur during *resting* respiration.

THE COUGH REFLEX

Neuroreceptors located in the **larynx** (voice box) and vocal cords, as well as in the trachea and large bronchi, can initiate a cough reflex when appropriately stimulated. Sudden increases in pressure in the thorax, inhaled chemical and physical agents, and endogenous (from within) substances such as **histamine** and certain **prostaglandins** cause coughing and, often, mucous secretion. It is obvious that coughing can be a symptom of many conditions, so it is important to avoid treating a cough symptomatically. The basic cause must be determined and resolved.

PANTING AND HOW IT COOLS

Dogs and a number of other animals pant when they are in hot environments; humans do not. On the other hand, humans have a relatively hairless body with abundant sweat glands and blood flow near the skin surface, aiding in control of their body temperature.

An interesting and useful physiological feature of the dog's respiratory system is a nasal gland that is capable of secreting great amounts of water, the evaporation of which is a major factor in cooling. Also, dogs have a mechanism that allows them to easily inhale via the nose and exhale via the mouth. It is not the case, as often believed, that evaporation from the dripping tongue is the way a dog loses heat. Despite its appearance, a panting dog is not breathing in and out of the mouth as is the case in mouth breathing in humans. The short-nosed dogs

Nasal Heat Loss

Measurements have shown that a panting dog forced to breath in and out of its mouth has an exhaled air temperature of about 29°C (degrees Centigrade). When allowed to inhale via its nose and exhale out of its mouth, the exhaled air measured 38°C, about the same as its body temperature. Using appropriate calculations, it can be shown that during the movement of one liter of air (about one quart), approximately fifteen calories of heat were lost during the first observation. However, when inhalation by nose and exhalation by mouth were allowed, the same amount of air movement resulted in the loss of nearly twenty-eight calories; the heat loss by this mechanism was nearly doubled. The amount of heat loss can be varied by changing the proportion of inhaled air that is discharged through the mouth. (Note: The calories referred to are 1/1,000 of the calories (kilocalories) commonly used in nutritional references.)

do not have the nasal anatomy required for optimal cooling with this mechanism.

As a dog becomes warm, panting begins, and the rate of panting is rather constant; it is a rate that is economical from an energy standpoint, and may be fifteen or more times the respiratory rate at rest. Only great stress causes the respiratory rate to increase. Instead of varying the rate of respiratory movement, dogs pant for a while and then cease panting for a period.

If panting is ordinarily at a constant rate, certain questions arise. How does the animal avoid upsetting the alveolar gas composition? How does a dog regulate the amount and effectiveness of the evaporation that takes place in the nasal cavity?

During panting, the amount of air moved with each breath is just a bit over the dead-space volume, that air filling the trachea and bronchi, and is breathed out again without having reached the alveoli. The end result is that a great volume of air movement occurs, but it is mostly dead-space air. The amount mixing with the air of the alveoli is only sufficient to maintain appropriate alveolar gas composition.

Experimental studies have shown that dogs at rest in cool environments may breath 100 percent in and out of their noses. However, the panting dog can vary the amount of the air that leaves (is exhaled) through the mouth—up to 100 percent leaving by way of the mouth. Because air inhaled through the nose picks up water by evaporation, the membranes of the nasal cavity and the blood that flows through them are cooled by the process. In a hot environment, it would not be expedient to exhale warm, humid air back out through the nose, heating its membranes during its outward passage. Thus, the heat loss is modulated by the proportion of inhaled air that is lost by way of the mouth. Sometimes, it is possible to hear the sound made by a panting dog when the air is redirected to exit through the mouth. This is much less visible than the wet tongue, but it is a remarkable and efficient system for losing body heat.

This system can be overloaded. In extreme environmental heat, a dog may not be able to *lose body heat* at a sufficient rate. If panting rate is driven too high, the control of gas composition is lost, and the amount of carbon dioxide lost increases as the alreolar air is diluted by excessive ventilation. This ultimately alters the blood pH, leading to respiratory **alkalosis** (an alkaline blood). This life-threatening condition is added to the rising body heat.

The principles just discussed are relevant to what happens when a dog is trapped in a closed automobile. Very soon, respiratory water loss will saturate the heated, trapped air and make evaporation ineffective. As body heat rapidly rises, excessive panting also leads to alkalosis, as mentioned. This lethal situation can occur quite rapidly, and *usually occurs because of a careless owner*. It is not at all a matter of merely using up the oxygen needed to sustain life.

NONRESPIRATORY LUNG FUNCTIONS

The blood that circulates through your dog's lungs can be affected in many ways in addition to gas exchange. Research has shown that large amounts of blood-borne **serotonin (5-hydroxytryptamine)** and **norepinephrine** are taken up by the lungs, which appears to act as a "filter" to remove such substances. Certain drugs (e.g., some antihistamines) are also taken out of the blood by tissues of the lung.

The lungs are confronted with an enormous amount of oxygen and could be damaged by it. The pulmonary capillary bed is especially exposed to damage by superoxide and other free radicals, and lethal injury can follow prolonged exposure to high oxygen levels. The capillary damage that can follow excessive oxygen exposure leads to pulmonary edema.

AGING AND THE RESPIRATORY SYSTEM

CHANGES IN THE CHEST WALL AND LUNGS

The chest wall becomes less elastic in old dogs because of calcification of cartilage in the joints where the ribs join the vertebrae. This calcification makes respiration difficult by requiring increased muscular effort. It also encourages a greater dependence on movement of the diaphragm to compensate for chest stiffness.

An overweight dog has an abdomen with fat deposits large enough to seriously oppose movement of the diaphragm. A general wasting of muscles during aging, including those for respiration, is added to all of the above factors. In fact, most aspects of respiratory fitness in your dog are altered during aging.

Cells that line the airways have cilia that aid in removing particulate material by "lifting" mucus up to the throat where it is unconsciously swallowed. This mechanism is reduced in effectiveness in the aged, and makes the respiratory system vulnerable to airborne infectious organisms. Also, **macrophages** (see the chapter The Protective Role of the Immune System) become less able to remove foreign material (including infectious organisms) deposited there, making the older dog more susceptible to respiratory infections and perhaps allowing small airway obstructions to accumulate.

RESPIRATION IN THE OLDER DOG

Alveolar ducts and enlargement of individual alveoli reduce the surface area relative to volume; the alveolar membranes also undergo thickening. A further handicap to gas exchange arises in the capillaries because of a **fibrosis** (abnormal fiber deposition) of their linings. It is not clear to what extent these changes are environmentally induced and how much are universal accompaniments of age although human cigarette smokers show these changes much more severely than nonsmokers of the same age.

A loss of lung elasticity requires more active effort to bring about expiration. In the aging lung, the relative inelasticity of small airways allows them to collapse fairly early in active expiration. This may bring about regional shunting of blood flow and interfere with alveolar-capillary exchange in the most susceptible areas of the lung.

Exercise

The advantages of exercise in slowing the age-related changes in respiratory function seem to be well established for humans. Because respiratory efficiency in the young adults allows activity at levels far above the resting state, preserving some of this reserve ability into older age should permit better health and activity levels.

It is speculation to claim that good respiratory function may extend life; there is no question that it will improve the quality of life and may aid in recovery from some diseases.

DISEASES OF THE RESPIRATORY SYSTEM

Respiratory diseases observed in elderly dogs may be primary, or they may be secondary to the reduction in pulmonary reserve that accompanies aging. Modern biomedical technology offers many useful treatments for respiratory disease; e.g., antibiotics for **tuberculosis** and **pneumonia**, early detection and therapy for lung cancer, pharmaceuticals for **asthma**, etc. However, several respiratory diseases are age-related or significantly serious in the aged.

BRACHYCEPHALIC AIRWAY SYNDROME

Short-nosed dogs, such as the Affenpinscher, Bulldog, Boxer, Boston Terrier, French Bulldog, Pug, Pekingese, and Shih Tzus, are commonly affected by **brachycephalic** (shortened head) **airway syndrome**. Their abnormal skulls have altered nasopharyngeal areas and nose anatomy, causing a restriction of air flow. Although present as inherited features at birth, problems may develop as such dogs grow older because of repeated infections and trauma. Of course, these breeds are considered less tolerant of heat stress and vigorous physical activity.

CHRONIC INFLAMMATORY RHINITIS

Chronic inflammatory rhinitis (inflammation of the mucous membranes of the nose) is seen in dogs, and is sometimes accompanied by **tonsillitis** (tonsil inflammation) or **pharyngitis** (inflammation of the pharynx). The symptoms vary widely, and your veterinarian must determine the cause and differentiate between several possible infections or the effects of tumors. Symptoms include a nasal discharge of long duration, sneezing spells, and gagging from postnasal drip. When dogs have had their immune systems impaired (e.g., after immuno-therapy or age-related immune dysfunction), other infections become more likely. Infections by certain fungi are especially difficult to manage.

VOCAL CORD PARALYSIS

Another condition that may impair respiration by blocking the larynx (voice box) is paralysis of the vocal cords; middle-aged and older dogs of the larger breeds seem most susceptible. Your veterinarian can distinguish this change in vocal quality from other voice changes and recommend the best care.

BRONCHIAL ASTHMA

Although uncommon in the dog, **bronchial asthma** is an allergic condition in which the smooth muscles of the airway contract, creating an impediment to free flow of air. This is especially so during exhalation, and a wheezing can usually be heard. Many substances may be agents of the allergic reaction, but grass seeds and pollen are the primary ones. Treatment with several drugs is possible, but severe cases may require steroids to control the pulmonary inflam-mation. Of course, careful veterinary observation is called for. As an asthmatic dog ages, the many bouts of asthma may lead to chronic lung disease and further compromise the older dog's well-being.

NASAL TUMORS

Tumors in the nasal cavity seem more common in dogs than in other domestic animals, and they occur in dogs that are usually over eight years of age.

The breeds that have been noted as being most susceptible are Airedale Terriers, Scottish Terriers, Basset Hounds, Old English Sheepdogs, Shetland Sheepdogs, Collies, and German Shorthaired Pointers. Several types of cancer are represented and some of them may spread (**metastasize**) to other tissues. As mentioned, symptoms may resemble those seen in rhinitis. Sometimes, facial deformity indicates the location and size of the tumor.

CANCER OF THE RESPIRATORY SYSTEM

Canine primary pulmonary neoplasia is rather rare, but may be increasing in frequency. It is distinctly age-related; the mean time of appearance has been reported as approximately ten years of age. Breed or sex association is not clearly evident.

This malignant tumor may develop in different parts of the lung and may metastasize to other lung areas. Depending upon the size and location of the tumors, symptoms may vary, but a long-lasting, nonproductive cough is the most common symptom. A loss of appetite, weight loss, and lethargy are other symptoms. When a large area of the lungs is involved, some breathing difficulty will be noticed, and the same is true when complications such as congestive heart failure also exist. As healthy lung tissue gives way to areas of damaged tissue, air may be released into the pleural space, producing a **pneumothorax**.

Treatment by surgery seems the only course of action. The advice of your veterinarian is extremely important in deciding how to pursue the care of a dog with lung cancer.

LUNG-RELATED PROBLEMS

Pleural Effusions (Fluid Pockets)

The formation of fluid pockets in the pleural space (**pleural effusions**) is not uncommon and may have various causes. The pleural space has a thin layer of fluid that serves as a lubricant between the two pleural membranes. A well-balanced mechanism governs the formation and control of this material. Blood pressure, plasma protein concentration, and the lymphatic system of drainage are components of this mechanism. Obviously, if any of these factors become abnormal, effusion of fluid into the pleural space may occur.

Because the lymph fluid (see the chapter The Cardiovascular System) is drained into a vein in the chest area, any damage to that drainage may result in the accumulation of lymph in the pleural space (**chylothorax**). Such damage may be caused by surgery or trauma to the chest, obstruction by tumors, or inflammation of the drainage duct.

Hemothorax is the term that indicates that blood has accumulated in the pleural space. Trauma, inadequate blood coagulation, and blockage of lung blood vessels by blood clots are among the things that participate in allowing blood to leak into this space. The veterinarian can reduce the blood that has accumulated by draining it out. However, the cause must be determined and controlled.

Other pleural effusions result from pleuritis (pleural infection), chest cancers, and congestive heart failure.

If a puncture wound of the chest or lung allows access of air to parts of the pleural space, air will enter and some lung areas will collapse because of their elastic property. Such a condition is referred to as a *pneumothorax*, but it need not cause a pleural effusion. The air is usually reabsorbed into the blood and body fluids in a relatively short time.

Lung Infections

Pneumonia may be caused by either bacterial or viral infection of the lungs, to which elderly dogs are more susceptible. Parasites, fungi, and yeasts also may infect lung tissue. Antibiotics, immunization, and modern medical management have reduced lung infections as causes of death of the elderly. Noninfectious causes of pneumonia include vascular insufficiency, aspiration of foreign substances, and lung injury by inhaled irritants.

Pulmonary tuberculosis is caused by a **mycobacterium** that is capable of infecting dogs, humans, and other animals; it multiplies slowly and may remain undetected for years before it is clinically evident. Many tissues may be infected, but the lungs are the major site. In past years, tuberculosis was epidemic among all ages of humans and a leading cause of death. The infection rate in dogs has declined as the human cases have become fewer. The decline in this disease has followed modern antibiotic use; however, it remains higher in the more susceptible older members of the population.

Distemper is caused by a virus; bacteria often invade, secondarily contributing to pneumonia. It is a serious respiratory infection usually seen in dogs only a few weeks old. However, this disease often creates damage that complicates the lives of older dogs. It has been estimated that about 50 percent of survivors of distemper develop neurological complications in later life. These include convulsions, oversensitivity (**hyperesthesia**), unsteady balance and gait, and exaggerated muscular jerking (**myoclonus**).

Parasite Infestation of the Lungs

The organism *Filaroides* (*Osterus*) *osleri* sometimes infests the lungs of dogs. Also, a lung fluke is found, which is contracted by eating infected snails, crayfish, or crabs. This fluke may infect humans as well. Parasites, by causing tissue injury and disruption of blood or air flow, may produce many of the symptoms of respiratory system disease discussed elsewhere in this chapter.

PULMONARY PROBLEMS

Pulmonary Obstructions

Chronic obstructive pulmonary disease (COPD) is a clear descriptive term for conditions in which pulmonary air movement is restricted. It is common in old dogs, and many causes are known. Besides infections that impair respiratory air movement over long periods of time, the most common conditions are chronic bronchitis (see under Coughing), chronic asthma (see under Bronchial Asthma), collapse of the trachea or bronchi, and fibrosis (excess tissue fiber deposits) of the airways. Because these are chronic conditions, continuous treatment is required. Complications caused by secondary pulmonary infections and other irritants are especially serious.

Chronic bronchitis is characterized by frequent coughing and considerable mucus production. Many irritants may cause this persistent condition. In the elderly, it is often coincident with other lung diseases such as chronic asthma.

Pulmonary Edema

Pulmonary edema *is not a disease; it is a manifestation of other malfunctions.* Commonly, it occurs when the left ventricle of the heart cannot accommodate the blood arriving to it by way of the pulmonary blood vessels. This is called *congestive heart failure.* This condition results in an increased capillary pressure in the lungs and an inappropriate filtration of fluid into the space around cells of the lung and into the alveoli (see the chapter The Cardiovascular System).

Infestation with heartworms may impede the pumping action of the heart or prevent proper closure of certain heart valves. Diseased heart valves alone can also produce this problem. This is discussed under Coughing below and also in the chapter The Cardiovascular System.

Another basis for pulmonary edema is an increased permeability of lung capillaries to plasma protein. Many conditions may bring about this change, e.g., **aspiration** (breathing into lungs) of gastric contents, inhalation of toxic fumes, and systemic or local infections. Even if infection is not a causal factor, pneumonia may develop later and contribute to the high mortality rate associated with the condition.

Because oxygen diffuses through membranes and water somewhat more rapidly than CO_2, the powerful stimulating action of carbon dioxide on the brain's respiratory center causes the heavy breathing seen when pulmonary edema exists.

COUGHING

Coughing may be symptomatic of many conditions. Allergies and diseases of the trachea, bronchi, or lungs, or their stimulation by internal or external irritants, may cause coughing. It is quite important to *recognize coughing that is a response to heart disease such as congestive heart failure, heartworms, or diseases of the heart valves*. In these conditions, the heart may be unable to effectively pump the blood that returns from the lungs. This allows the pressure in the lung circulation to "back up," bringing about pulmonary edema (see above and the chapter The Cardiovascular System). The fluid accumulating in the lungs impairs gas exchange and stimulates coughing.

Kennel cough (**tracheobronchitis**) is an infection caused by **para-influenza virus, canine adenovirus**, or, sometimes, distemper virus combined with a bacterium (*Bordetella*). It is highly contagious and the stress of kennel conditions may predispose to it. A dry, spasmodic cough appears five to ten days after exposure to the infecting organisms. It is usually self-limiting in otherwise healthy dogs, but older dogs and puppies will not tolerate it as well. Lung inflammation caused by several parasites may lead to secondary infection. Vaccines are available for most of the infectious agents.

Dogs over five years of age, especially individuals in the small breeds (e.g., Toy Poodles, Yorkshire Terriers, Chihuahuas, and Pomeranians), and particularly those that are obese, may suffer **canine chronic bronchitis**. Coughing is a notable feature. Although the cause or causes of this serious and distressing condition are not understood, several factors, including some infections, are considered. Acute bronchitis, caused by a number of different infectious organisms, may alter the function of the cells lining the bronchi so that mucus is not effectively lifted out of the respiratory tree, and this may persist for years after the infection.

Otherwise unnoticed pollutants (e.g., cigarette smoke, sulfur dioxide fumes, and other environmental factors) are also suspected agents. In some cases, allergies are thought to be causal, including allergies to some parasites.

Chronic bronchitis presents your veterinarian with a challenging condition because there seems to be no specific treatment. Avoiding environmental pollutants (especially cigarette smoke), losing excess weight, maintaining good hydration so that mucus is less thick, and avoiding excess physical activity are reasonable actions. Certain drugs that dilate the respiratory pathways (**bron-chodilators**) act on the brain to suppress the cough reflex; others have antihistamine effects that may be helpful; steroids seem indicated in the worst cases. Unfortunately, some dogs may not be relieved to the extent desired.

When a dog has lung cancer, coughing may be the only symptom noticed at first. Cancer of the lung may be primary to the lung, or secondary if it has spread there from cancer elsewhere in the body. Your veterinarian will determine if surgery and chemotherapy are appropriate in each case.

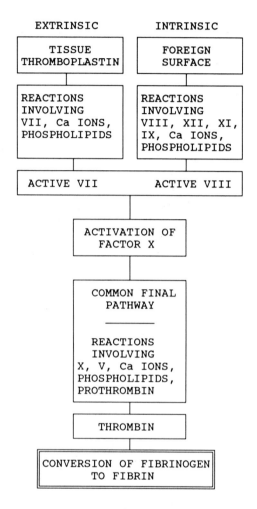

Clotting of Blood Blood clotting results from the conversion of fibrinogen to fibrin. This may occur in the body or after blood is outside of the vascular and tissue spaces. When clotting is initiated within the body, the series of reactions are said to be intrinsic; it is important to have an intrinsic system for clotting in order to stop blood loss at small injury sites. Massive injuries may invoke both intrinsic and extrinsic reaction paths.

12

The Blood and
Body Fluids:
Distribution and Control

INTRODUCTION TO FUNCTIONS AND PROPERTIES OF THE BLOOD

The blood and body fluids have often been referred to as "the sea within us," an analogy to the stable, seawater environment in which cells first evolved. This viewpoint is in keeping with the many functions served by the blood: respiratory, nutritive, excretory, protective, and regulatory.

The first attempts to transfuse blood into humans was disastrous because animal bloods were used. Because the principles of incompatibility between bloods were not known, even the first attempts to transfuse with human blood fared little better. It was not until early in this century, following discovery of blood groups and anticoagulant agents, that transfusion became successful. It is now practical in both human and veterinary medicine. The different blood groups in animal species show unique patterns for each individual.

Blood has several cell populations (Table 12.1). They are generally classified as red blood cells (**erythrocytes**) and white blood cells (**leukocytes**). Subgroups of the latter will be discussed below and in the chapter The Protective Role of the Immune System. Other particulate elements of the blood are the small **blood platelets** and **chylomicrons** (fat droplets).

Plasma is the fluid portion of blood. It is a water solution made up of many

TABLE 12.1　Cells and Particles of the Blood

ERYTHROCYTES

PLATELETS

LEUKOCYTES
　Granulocytes
　　Neutrophils
　　Basophils
　　Eosinophils
　Agranulocytes
　　Monocytes
　　Lymphocytes

substances, including electrolytes, nutritive and waste material, hormones and other regulatory agents, and various plasma proteins. When blood clots form, the plasma protein **fibrinogen** is converted into an insoluble polymer, **fibrin**, which traps the formed elements, leaving a straw-colored, cell-free fluid called **serum**.

All blood cells arise by multiplication and differentiation from **pluripotent stem cells**, primarily in the **bone marrow**. The sequences of these processes is given in detail in the chapter The Protective Role of the Immune System.

WHITE BLOOD CELLS (LEUKOCYTES)

The population of cells called leukocytes (white blood cells or WBCs) are varied in type, and their immunological and regulatory functions are described in the chapter The Protective Role of the Immune System. Some are involved in production of antibodies, while others recognize foreign cells and abnormal cells, mounting cell-mediated attacks against them. All of these types have their primary origin in the bone marrow. White blood cells are larger and more spherical than the rather flat red blood cells; they often meet considerable resistance in passing through smaller blood vessels.

Neutrophils, named because their cytoplasmic granules stain with neutral dyes, normally make up about 65 percent of the population of leukocytes. White blood cells are attracted to injured areas on blood vessel walls, and neutrophils readily pass through the wall into the tissue spaces. They pass between cells of blood vessel walls by inserting a **pseudopod** (false foot) between cells and "flowing" through. Once in an area of infection, neutrophils ingest bacteria and other particulate material.

Basophils (their cytoplasmic granules stain with basic dyes) and **eosinophils** (their cytoplasmic granules stain with eosin dyes), along with neutrophils, constitute the cells of the group called **granulocytes** simply because of granules that are present in the cytoplasm of all of them. Such classification is based on their anatomy, not their function. Basophils, less than 1 percent of white blood cells, contain histamine in their granules. The release of this histamine characterizes allergic reactions. Eosinophils are often found outside of the blood, especially in the bowel wall, lungs, and skin. They increase in number during parasite infections and with allergic reactions.

Monocytes are the largest white blood cells and are about 5 percent of the leukocytes. Monocytes are transformed into large, fixed **macrophages** and participate in the phagocytic removal of infectious organisms.

Lymphocytes, have rather clear, granule-free cytoplasm and are called **agranulocytes** (without granules). However, the roles of lymphocytes are quite different from the other leukocytes. Those known as **B lymphocytes** produce antibodies. **T lymphocytes** are varied and their functions include immune activity against viruses as well as bacteria.

Collectively, lymphocytes control much immune activity and are the principals in what is known as **cellular immunity**, the types of reactions that result in foreign tissue rejection or, sometimes, attacks against cancer cells. Lymphocytes normally are 20 to 25 percent of all white blood cells.

Whenever the number of leukocytes in the blood is below a normal range, **leukocytopenia** is said to exist. An excess number of leukocytes in the blood is known as **leukocytosis**. An increase in leukocyte concentration can be a response to infection, allergy, or a cancer of leukocyte-producing tissue.

BLOOD PLATELETS

Blood platelets are also known as **thrombocytes** (blood-clot cells); they are not true cells. Fragments of larger cells, platelets are much smaller than red blood cells. They are important in initiating the clotting of blood, and they participate in other processes that maintain intact blood vessels. They aggregate at sites of blood vessel injury, block small breaks, and facilitate clotting in larger injuries. Platelets have a life span of only a few days and must be actively produced to maintain a normal blood concentration.

RED BLOOD CELLS (ERYTHROCYTES)

Red blood cells (erythrocytes) are well known for their participation in oxygen and carbon dioxide transport in the blood, making obvious the need for adequate iron intake for **hemoglobin** (see the chapters The Respiratory System and Nutrition and Metabolism). They arise from **pluripotent** cells (cells able to give rise to several types of cells) in the bone marrow. The normal level of red blood cells in dog's blood is 5 to 9 million per cubic millimeter; this is somewhat higher and more variable than in humans. A low level of red blood cells (RBCs) or the hemoglobin in them is known as **anemia**.

Erythropoiesis (red cell production) requires an adequate intake of vitamins B_{12} and folic acid (folacin), as well as protein and iron (see the chapter Nutrition and Metabolism). Lack of either vitamin B_{12} or folic acid results in a delay in the release of red blood cells from the bone marrow; the effect is production of fewer, but larger than normal, erythrocytes. Vitamin B_{12} deficiency leads to the condition referred to as **pernicious anemia** in humans. However, nutritional anemias are rare in dogs that are maintained on the good diets that are currently available (see under Anemia).

Erythrocyte production in the bone marrow is controlled by **erythropoietin**, a hormone produced by the kidney (see the chapters The Endocrine System and The Urinary System). Bone marrow has a substantial reserve capacity for RBC production; after blood loss by hemorrhage or following red blood cell destruction, the production rate may rise to several times normal.

Erythrocytes have a finite life span; changes take place in them as they age and make them subject to removal by the spleen and liver. They are removed from the blood when they are about 120 days old in humans and at a similar age in dogs. The fact that they lose their nuclei in the course of differentiation from their stem cells makes it impossible for them to reproduce themselves; they are renewed by differentiation of bone marrow stem cells. Hemoglobin is synthesized in the differentiating red blood cell.

When aged red blood cells are destroyed in the spleen or liver, the protein and fat portions are returned to the metabolic pools of the body for reuse in general metabolism. The iron is removed from the heme of hemoglobin, and it is almost quantitatively conserved for reuse. The remaining heme material is converted into a colored substance, **bilirubin** (a **bile pigment**), and excreted into the intestine with the bile. Some of the bilirubin is further modified in the intestine, reabsorbed, and excreted in the urine, contributing to urine color. In certain liver diseases, the excretion of bile pigment is faulty; bilirubin then accumulates in the blood and gives rise to **jaundice**, a yellow appearance that can be noticed in the **sclera** of a dog's eyes.

Anemia may be the consequence of blood cell loss, bone marrow failure from various causes, immune or chemical injury to RBCs, lack of adequate iron or other nutrient needs, and sometimes from an abnormal function of the spleen (**hypersplenism**) that causes it to prematurely remove red blood cells from circulation.

The surface membrane of red blood cells contains genetically determined molecules known as **antigens** that are able to react with antibodies (see the chapter The Protective Role of the Immune System). It has been shown that dogs have seven or eight major blood group systems. Antibodies (**isoagglutinins**) that react with some red blood cell antigens (immune counterparts of antibodies) occur naturally in the blood of dogs. These seem related to the A antigens of the human ABO blood group system. Other erythrocyte antigens in the dog have no corresponding antibodies unless a dog has been exposed to antigens absent in itself. Pregnancy, with a fetus possessing an antigen not present in its mother, may cause her to develop antibodies to that blood group factor. Also, repeated transfusions or immunization with vaccines containing dog blood products may induce blood group factor antibodies in susceptible dogs.

Typing of a dog's blood is useful when transfusions are contemplated. Also, the genetic profile related to a dog's blood groups may be useful when challenging breeding misalliances from natural mating, artificial insemination, or embryo transfers. However, knowledge of the antigens that are associated with leukocytes, **HLA antigens**, may be more useful for some of these situations in dogs (see the chapter The Protective Role of the Immune System).

KEEPING BLOOD WITHIN THE BLOOD VESSELS (HEMOSTASIS)

The term **hemostasis** alludes to prevention of bleeding. Blood clotting is the most evident means of plugging leaks in the vascular system, but other mechanisms are important. For example, blood platelets react by becoming "sticky" and gathering at injury sites, resulting in a mechanical blockage if the hole is small enough. Along with platelet gathering, the exposed collagen in blood vessel walls contracts and brings about contraction of broken surfaces on small blood vessels. Platelets release a number of chemical agents that enhance platelet adherence, stimulate local vasoconstriction, and some platelet substances participate in the formation of blood clots.

A substance produced by endothelial cells lining blood vessels, **von Ville-brand factor**, is also needed to promote this platelet adhesion.

Historically, many terms have been assigned to the numerous substances that participate in clotting. Hereafter, the generally accepted Roman numeral

---

Blood Clotting—Extrinsic and Intrinsic

Extrinsic clotting is initiated by tissue injury, the release of some type of tissue factor (a *thromboplastin*), and its reaction with one of the enzymes involved in the clotting sequence. *Intrinsic clotting* involves a somewhat different series of reactions; it occurs when *factor XII* contacts a foreign surface. These reactions have been aptly called a "cascade of enzymes" because most of the reagents are enzymes, and each, as it is activated, activates another in turn.

In extrinsic clotting, damaged tissue releases a *tissue factor* that initiates reactions between several other substances present in the blood (factors VII, X, V, calcium ions, and specific *phospholipids*) to produce a *thromboplastic* substance, a substance that is able to convert factor II (*prothrombin*) to *thrombin.* The clotting process is finalized when thrombin converts factor I (*fibrinogen*) to *fibrin*, and a *polymer* (a linkage of many molecules) of fibrin forms.

When blood clots form within a few minutes after the blood contacts negatively charged foreign surfaces, such as glass or collagen molecules, intrinsic clotting takes place. In this case, the effect of surface contact and the release of specific phospholipids from platelets participate in reactions that include factors XII, XI, IX, VII, X, V, and calcium ions to produce a thromboplastin. Factor VII is known as *antihemophilic factor*; it is absent from the blood of *hemophiliacs* because of a genetic defect, but it may be extracted from normal blood to be administered to dogs with hemophilia.

---

designations for these factors will be used, sometimes with common terms, to avoid the confusion of many synonyms (see Table 12.2). The accompanying sidebar briefly provides details of extrinsic and intrinsic clotting of blood.

The vascular system would be impaired by the failure of blood to remain fluid. To help prevent such failure, the body produces an enzyme called **plasmin**, which has the ability to split fibrin molecules (in a process called **fibrinolysis**) as well as some other molecules that participate in the clotting process. Thus, it acts as an inhibitor to clotting, and, if clotting occurs, it causes the clot to dissolve after a time. Substances that dissolve clots are now a significant part of medicine; **streptokinase**, **urokinase**, and tissue-type plasminogen activator (t-PA) are enzymes now available to be used to break up clots that have already formed.

Anticoagulants

Heparin, produced by the liver, is a powerful anticoagulant. Other anticlotting agents also exist. These factors participate in a coagulation/anticoagulation equilibrium—a steady state in the blood. When intravascular clotting is known to be a risk, as during cardiovascular surgery, heparin (an **antithrombin**) may be infused until the risk subsides.

Another protection against uncontrolled clotting is the production of a **prostaglandin** derivative, **prostacyclin**, by the normal endothelial lining of blood vessels. This appears to prevent platelets from sticking to normal vessel walls and to one another. It has been learned that aspirin may be administered in small doses to impair platelet production of the prostaglandin derivative **thromboxane A**, which promotes platelet aggregation. *You should never repeatedly administer aspirin to a dog without a veterinarian's advice because it is capable of causing many undesirable effects in inappropriate doses.*

In some cases, drugs of the coumarin group (i.e., dicoumarol, Warfarin) may be administered to lower excessive coagulability in dogs. The coumarins interfere with the liver's synthesis of prothrombin by competing with the action

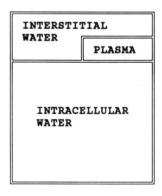

Body Water Compartments It is convenient to view the water of the body as being either intracellular or extracellular. The latter can be further divided into that between cells (interstitial) and that in the blood plasma. Intracellular water is clearly the largest volume.

of vitamin K. Warfarin and similar compounds are found in popular rodent poisons; a serious blood clotting deficit develops when rodents (or dogs) consume them regularly. However, it is important to note that newer substances that interfere with vitamin K have been developed that have profound effects long after a single ingestion.

BODY FLUIDS

The water of the body is viewed as occupying various compartments. The principal division is between **intracellular** and **extracellular** compartments; the extracellular volume includes the blood plasma volume and the space about extravascular cells, the **interstitial fluid**. In a healthy adult dog, the total body water is about 70 percent of the body weight; half of this is inside cells.

A measurement of whole blood volume must take into account the cells of the blood. This is done by centrifuging (spinning) a blood sample and determining the **hematocrit**, the percentage of the packed cells in whole blood. The whole blood volume is usually about 90 ml per kilogram of body weight when measured in a healthy dog.

The composition of plasma is well regulated in a healthy dog. Many electrolytes (bicarbonate, calcium, potassium, sodium, and chloride ions) are present in milligram quantities per 100 ml of plasma. These are important amounts since they play vital roles in the osmotic pressure balance between the inside and outside of cells, in addition to their metabolic roles. Similarly, small amounts of hormones, glucose, and urea are present. They are major factors in

TABLE 12.2   Designation of Blood Clotting Factors

Factor	Name
I	Fibrinogen
Enzyme activity	
II	Prothrombin
VII	Proconvertin
IX	Plasma thromboplastin component; Christmas factor
X	Stuart-Prower factor
XI	Plasma thromboplastin antecedent
XII	Hageman factor
Cofactor activity	
III	Tissue thromboplastin
IV	Calcium ions
V	Proaccelerin
VIII	Antihemophilic factor.

osmotically "holding" water in the intracellular and extracellular compartments that have been discussed.

On the other hand, the loss of electrolytes, especially sodium, reduces the whole extracellular compartment; however, this volume loss in the plasma compartment also reduces blood pressure. The use of diuretics to cause sodium loss in order to lower blood pressure in hypertension is discussed in the chapter The Urinary System.

Electrolytes are also crucial in maintaining the pH (acidity/alkalinity) of the blood, which must be kept in the range of 7.35 to 7.45— *neutral is 7.0*. This is primarily accomplished by the kidneys and lungs, with contributions by the intestinal tract. When pH changes, the acid-base environment is no longer optimal for enzyme function. *The effect of pH on excitable tissue is very important;* **acidosis** *or* **alkalosis** *will impair nerve condition and heart contraction.* Electrolyte levels and the ratio between some of them (e.g., calcium and potassium) also affect excitable tissue.

AGING BLOOD CELLS

It has been mentioned that a dog's red blood cells have a life span reported to be in the range of 90 to 135 days. As they age, they become more dense and more fragile, and they lose potassium. Both mechanical stress and exposure to osmotic extremes result in damage more readily as they age. These changes are related to the red blood cell's age, not the age of the dog.

However, when erythrocytes from elderly individuals are placed in salt solutions of low concentration (**hypotonic** solutions), they **hemolyze** (swell and rupture) more readily than those from younger animals. Additionally, an older animal's erythrocytes have a somewhat greater diameter and volume.

Individual red blood cells that are near the end of their life are removed by lymphoid tissue, especially the spleen. Changes in these tissues in older animals may leave some of these fragile cells in the circulation a little longer. Yet, according to some studies, red cell life span seems unchanged in the elderly.

The volume of bone marrow that is capable of red blood cell production is reduced in the aged, at least in the human. This reduction compromises the speed of red blood cell production when it must correct an anemia because of hemorrhage or erythrocyte destruction, but not the ultimate capacity to restore a normal RBC count at a slower rate.

No evidence suggests functional alterations in the blood platelets of the aged. However, variable changes occur in the coagulation factors XI, XII, and a natural antithrombin activity.

Simple measurements, such as a white blood cell count, do not reveal age-related changes in the animals that have been studied. However, changes in specific categories of cells may be evident, and changes in their functional properties may be important. A significant age-related increase in B lymphocytes has been reported. Granulocytes show some anatomical changes in the appearance of their cell nuclei.

BLOOD PLASMA COMPOSITION IN THE AGED DOG

A characteristic fall in albumin concentration with age results in a lowered osmotic pressure across capillary walls. This lowered osmotic pressure causes the formation of **edema** and **ascites** (abdominal fluid).

The progressive, age-related loss of renal function results in higher levels of wastes in the blood: urea, uric acid, creatinine, etc. The total electrolyte concentration is maintained, but changes in individual electrolyte levels occur. Bicarbonate levels fall, and there may be a slight fall in blood calcium and phosphate levels.

DISEASES RELATED TO BLOOD AND BODY FLUIDS

Although changes in the blood and body fluids are not particularly noticeable in the healthy aged, diseases of many of the body's systems alter these fluids and related cells.

BODY FLUIDS AND DISEASE

The body fluids are not the origin of primary disease, but they commonly show the effects of many diseases.

For example, an increase in body water may be the result of the kidneys' failure to excrete it. A reduction in body water may be the result of the loss of blood by hemorrhage or the loss of water in diarrhea and vomiting. Abnormal plasma protein levels can allow water to leave the blood and accumulate in tissue spaces (edema). Loss of fluid through respiration is often overlooked; it can be critical for an older dog, especially when it is suffering a serious illness.

When blood loss by hemorrhage is great, the blood pressure may fall and the circulation fail (see the chapter The Cardiovascular System). This is **cardiovascular shock** and demands immediate veterinary attention. If the hemorrhage is less severe, the blood volume may be returned to near normal by osmotic forces drawing fluid into the capillary blood. Blood transfusion is the accepted treatment for blood loss, although rehydration by drinking water or prescribed solutions may be appropriate in less severe cases.

ANEMIA

Anemia is discussed in several connections in this chapter and in the chapters The Respiratory System and Nutrition and Metabolism. In addition to acute hemorrhage, it may be caused by loss of blood from ulcers and wounds, depression of bone marrow, and destruction of red blood cells. Bone marrow depression, which may affect both red and white blood cell production, may be the result of chronic use of some medications and exposure to environmental toxins. There is good reason to discuss the effects of medication in use with your veterinarian if your dog is found to have anemia. Kidney disease may occasionally be responsible for failure to produce erythropoietin.

DISEASES AND THE WHITE BLOOD CELLS

Because of their role in immunity, important additional information on white blood cells will be found in the chapter The Protective Role of the Immune System.

Neutrophilia is not a disease; it is the condition in which the blood level of *neutrophils* is *higher* than normal. A high neutrophil count may be a response to infections. Neutrophilia is also associated with diseases that have an immune relationship, such as **autoimmune hemolytic anemia**, **lupus erythematosus**, and **rheumatoid arthritis**. Tissue damage caused by burns, blocked blood flow, or cancer may result in increased neutrophils. The administration of corticosteroids and a reaction to fear and excitement may also induce neutrophilia.

Neutropenia, a *low level of neutrophils*, commonly reflects a bone marrow depression of cell production. **Canine parvovirus** infection is one of the infections known to suppress bone marrow. If the neutrophils are low, the dog is more susceptible to infections. A number of drugs suppress the bone marrow and cause neutropenia as well as anemia. Among these are high estrogens and cancer chemotherapy drugs.

Lymphocytosis (excess lymphocytes) follows fear and excitement, certain infections, and cancers of the lymphoid tissue. Its opposite, **lymphopenia**, a deficiency of lymphocytes, occurs in infections such as **parvoviral enteritis**, **canine distemper**, **coronaviral enteritis**, and **infectious canine hepatitis**. Corticosteroids may produce lymphopenia, as can immunosuppressive drugs and X-radiation. A number of conditions, such as inflammation of the intestinal wall (**enteritis**), may cause a loss of the lymph fluid and the lymphocytes in it.

Eosinophilia (increased eosinophils) is notable in dogs infected with various parasites, especially **nematodes** (worms). When fleas and ticks are to blame, the mechanism is probably associated with allergic reactions. Hypersensitivity or inflammatory reactions of a number of tissues are reported to be associated with eosinophilia, and a few cancers seem to produce it.

Dogs with heartworms and hookworms show **basophilia** (increased number of basophils). The response of basophils resembles that of eosinophils. It has been reported in association with other parasites, the types of sensitivities that involve eosinophils, drugs such as heparin and penicillin, and cancer of the basophil stem cell line.

The **leukemias** and **myeloproliferative** conditions show increased white blood cells, as expected. These are malignancies of the cell lines in the bone marrow that produce white blood cells. Sustained cell division is characteristic of cancer. Leukemia in the dog is seen often by the veterinarian, but it is much more frequent in cats.

The leukemia most often seen in dogs is **lymphoid leukemia**. The symptoms are variable, but they usually include the nonspecific signs of lethargy, loss of appetite, loss of weight, fever, vomiting, and diarrhea. Your veterinarian will seek more specific signs.

BLOOD CLOTS IN BLOOD VESSELS (HEMOSTATIC FAILURES)

Thrombocytopenia (lowered blood platelet count) may cause failure of the hemostatic system by predisposing to abnormal bleeding into tissues. Platelets may be removed from the blood at a rate above normal.

Thrombocytopenia is the most common hemorrhagic disease (disease with excessive bleeding) in the dog. It may result from bone marrow suppression with leukemia or bone marrow failure caused by certain drugs, including many of the medicines used for therapy of other diseases, e.g., antibiotics and anti-inflammatory agents. Considerable exposure to X rays will suppress most bone marrow functions, including platelet production.

A **thrombus** is a blood clot in the heart or arteries (rarely in the general veins of dogs). If all or a portion of the clot breaks away and travels to another site, it is called an **embolus**. Infection of the heart lining (**endocarditis**) may initiate a thrombus. Heartworm infection in dogs may lead to thrombi in the right atrium and in the veins where they enter the right atrium. Emboli from these clots can gain access to the arteries leading into the lungs, causing **pulmonary thromboembolic** (PTE) **disease**. In conditions such as these, your veterinarian may use carefully chosen doses of aspirin and other antiplatelet drugs.

Antithrombins, normally present in the blood, help prevent runaway clotting. In one study of a purebred Beagle colony, twenty of the fifty-two dogs examined that had glomerular disease also showed evidence of thrombosis. The damaged glomeruli leak several plasma proteins into the urine, including **antithrombin III**. Dogs with liver failure may fail to produce most of the coagulation factors, as well as antithrombin III. However, they are less likely to have severe thrombosis because they have lost the coagulation factors themselves.

BLOOD COAGULATION AND CANCER

Blood platelets are abnormal in animals with a number of types of cancer. If the associated tumors are successfully treated, platelets return to normal. In tumor-bearing dogs, the platelet life span may be shortened. Numbers of platelets may be reduced and their functions may be altered. Also, platelets have been shown to be involved in the spread of cancer (metastasis).

Lymphosarcoma and acute leukemia diminish platelet production, along with other marrow-derived cells. Other malignancies may metastasize to the marrow and displace normal marrow cells.

Estrogens (see the chapters The Endocrine System and The Reproductive System) in large amounts suppress bone marrow in dogs, resulting in lower production of marrow-derived cells. Tumors of **Sertoli** cells (cells in the male's testes) are known to produce estrogens. Studies of these tumors in dogs have shown that tumors in undescended testes are primarily involved. Similarly, some ovarian tumors in bitches produce excessive estrogens.

For reasons not yet understood, some dogs with bone marrow cancer, and other tumors, will develop destructive antibodies against blood platelets. Also, dogs with cancer sometimes produce platelets that have a reduced survival time in the bloodstream. Advanced lymphosarcoma and metastasized **adenocarcinoma** are notable in this association. Also, platelet numbers may be low because they have been used up in the persistent clotting throughout the body.

Thrombocytosis (above-normal platelet count) is seen in some dogs with cancers. A mechanism for this association is not known.

In addition to the association of cancer and platelet abnormality, alterations occur in the blood's coagulation factors. The cancer may alter liver and other functions to bring this about. However, cancer chemotherapy and the damage to various organ functions by a primary tumor are two other causes of blood coagulation abnormalities. These are complex clinical problems, calling for the exercise of substantial knowledge by your veterinarian.

DISSEMINATED INTRAVASCULAR COAGULATION

One of the most common disorders of coagulation in dogs is called **disseminated intravascular coagulation** (DIC). It is not a disease in itself; it is a condition caused by some underlying disease that coincidentally overwhelms the ordinarily prevented blood clotting within blood vessels. It is a very serious condition and often marks the terminal phase of deadly illnesses.

Because DIC is secondary to other conditions, treating the underlying condition is important. However, blood transfusions may be life-saving if restoring normal clotting mechanisms prevents abnormal bleeding and shock.

CANINE VON VILLEBRAND DISEASE

Reports of von Villebrand disease in dogs, pigs, rabbits, and humans have been made. About thirty dog breeds have signs of this genetically transmitted disease. The characteristic bleeding tendency is caused by the failure of blood platelets to form a normal platelet plug at sites of blood vessel injury.

Canine von Villebrand disease was first reported in a Scottish Terrier. Subsequently, Chesapeake Bay Retrievers, Doberman Pinschers, Airedale Terriers, and German Shorthaired Pointers have been studied closely. In fact, certain veterinary colleges have established families of affected dogs in order to learn how it is inherited, how it should be diagnosed, and how it should be treated. It varies in severity between different groups, e.g., Doberman Pinschers have a more severe form than Airedale Terriers. Whether a dog with von Villebrand disease will survive injuries, surgeries, etc., and reach old age may depend on the type inherited and the veterinary care given it.

The endothelial cells that line blood vessels have been shown to produce von Villebrand factor, a factor needed for platelets to adhere to blood vessel walls and one another. Also, this factor stabilizes factor VII, the blood factor missing in dogs with hemophilia.

In pregnant bitches, von Villebrand factor increases at the time of delivery. Sometimes, liver disease and bacterial toxins cause increases in von Villebrand factor. Clinical symptoms of the disease include blood in the urine, bleeding gums, and bloody diarrhea. Excessive bleeding while giving birth or during any surgical procedure, including toenail trimming, is a concern. Your veterinarian will be familiar with the many other conditions and signs associated with von Villebrand disease.

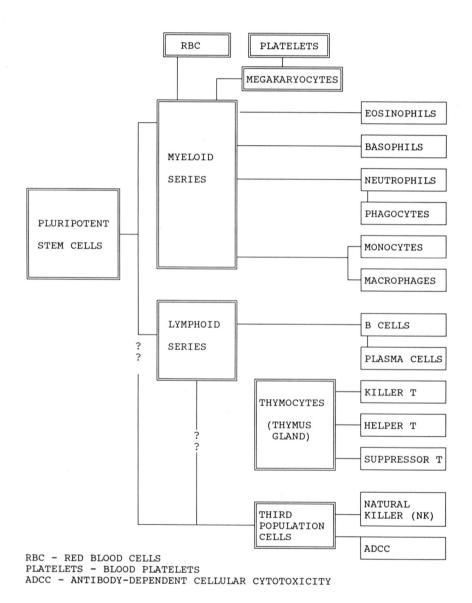

RBC - RED BLOOD CELLS
PLATELETS - BLOOD PLATELETS
ADCC - ANTIBODY-DEPENDENT CELLULAR CYTOTOXICITY

Cells of the Immune System This diagram illustrates the origin and relationships between cells of the immune system.

13

The Protective Role
of the Immune System

THE MEANING OF IMMUNITY

In common thought, *immune* implies that an individual cannot be hurt by an event; i.e., one is "immune" to danger. Scientists use the term to indicate a biological response that usually results in a protective reaction. However, some immune responses are part of allergic reactions.

Even earthworms are able to immunologically reject body wall transplants from genetically distant donors. Other **invertebrate** (without backbone) animals have wandering cells that are able to **phagocytose** (engulf) foreign material that might injure or infect the host. Thus, the immune system is quite old from an evolutionary standpoint.

The immune processes may fall into either of two categories: **innate** mechanisms and **adaptive** mechanisms. The innate system is generally always present to prevent or contain infection. Adaptive mechanisms establish a system of recognition so that future infections by the same agents will initiate a more prompt, effective defense. The adaptive system has its own features and also uses many elements of the innate system.

Certain cells of the immune system recognize the differences between cells of the self and those that are nonself. This ability permits an **immune surveillance system** that detects cells that have undergone change, perhaps by becoming cancerous. This system blocks efforts to surgically replace diseased organs and tissues by transplantation from genetically different donors. **Autoimmunity** is the failure of this recognition function; cells of the self are perceived as foreign.

Genetic factors play significant roles in immunity. The cells of the immune system may change; they may not recognize appropriate targets, or they may fail to respond effectively. The elderly regularly show differences in nearly all immune functions that have been studied. Many age-related changes occur during the first quarter of the life span, not just the later years. This system is dynamic in its function at any age and in the progression of its changes throughout life.

AN OVERVIEW OF THE IMMUNE SYSTEM

The bone marrow contains **stem cells**, which produce many types of cells of the immune system. These stem cells are also the source of red blood cells, which carry oxygen and are not immune cells, and blood platelets, which initiate and take part in blood clotting.

The cells that arise from stem cell differentiation are classified as **myeloid series** and **lymphoid series**. This is a classification based on cell origin. The myeloid series includes red blood cells, **megakaryocytes** (bone marrow cells that give rise to blood platelets), and immune cells. Myeloid white blood cells include the **neutrophils**, the most abundant of all the white blood cells. Another myeloid cell, the **monocyte**, is a cell with a single, uniform nucleus. **Eosinophils** are involved in immune activity against parasitic organisms and some allergies. **Basophils** contain **heparin** (an anticoagulant), a factor that attracts eosinophils, and the **histamine** involved in allergy. **Mast cells**, fixed cells outside the blood, are closely related to basophils and release a considerable amount of histamine in certain reactions. Histamine causes dilation of small blood vessels and permits greater permeability of their walls. This enhances local blood flow and access by immune system reagents. It also participates in allergic reactions.

The lymphoid series of white blood cells consists of the several types of **lymphocytes**. All of these originate in the bone marrow and further differentiate into subtypes. The **B lymphocytes** (B cells) give rise to antibody-producing **plasma cells** found in **lymphoid** organs (e.g., lymph nodes) and other tissue. Immature lymphocytes that pass through the **thymus gland** are stimulated to become **T lymphocytes** (T cells) belonging to one of at least three classes: **cytotoxic T cells** (killer T cells), which directly kill target cells; **helper T lymphocytes** (helper T cells), which play several roles in coordinating immune activity; or **suppressor T lymphocytes** (suppressor T cells), which normally regulate the orderly cessation of an immune response.

Antibodies (**immunoglobulins**—Ig) are glycoproteins that are produced in direct response to many substances. The material that stimulates antibody production is called an **antigen** and its antibody is quite specific for it. Reaction with an antibody may damage the antigen or identify it to immune cells. The different types of antibodies have various functions (see sidebar).

Antibodies—Classes and Functions

There are several classes of *antibodies* (also known as *immunoglobulins*—Ig); they are designated as IgG, IgA, IgM, IgD, and IgE. IgG is the predominant antibody, constituting about three-quarters of all antibodies in the blood and extravascular fluid. It is the main antibody of the *secondary immune response*, and IgG includes a class of antibody (antitoxin) that reacts with molecular toxins.

Infectious organisms with complex *antigens* (the molecules that induce specific antibody synthesis) stimulate early production of IgM; it is primarily found in the blood, representing about 10 % of antibodies there.

IgA makes up 15 to 20 % of antibodies in the blood. However, it is found abundantly in body secretions (and known as *secretory IgA*) such as saliva, secretions of the lung passageways (*tracheobronchial secretions*), *colostrum* (early secretions from the breasts), milk, and secretions of the *genitourinary system*.

The function of the small amount of IgD that is found in the blood is not clear; it is abundant in the membranes of *B lymphocytes* where it may participate in the differentiation of these cells.

IgE is found on the surfaces of blood-borne *basophils* and the surfaces of basophil-derived *mast cells*, which are fixed-position cells throughout the body's tissues. Both of these cells contain *histamine*, which is a potent *vasodilator*, but it also stimulates some smooth muscle cells, e.g., those in the trachea. IgE appears to be active in the body's defense against *helminth* (worm) parasites. Unfortunately, IgE reacts with antigenic materials that are responsible for the hypersensitivity seen in conditions such as *asthma* and *allergies*.

INNATE IMMUNE MECHANISMS

When a microorganism attempts to grow in the tissues of the body, the condition is considered an **infection**. An infecting organism must first break such barriers as (1) the skin; (2) secretions of the **sebaceous glands** (skin glands); (3) **mucus** discharge from mouth, anus, and nose; (4) the action of **cilia** (fine hairs) of the windpipe lining that move particles out of the lung; (5) the stomach's acid; (6) normal organisms that live in harmony with the tissues of the vagina and intestines but compete with organisms capable of infecting; (7) **spermine** found in semen of the male; (8) or the very important bactericidal enzyme **lysozyme** found in tears of the eyes and many other body secretions, and which damages the membranes of bacteria.

If an infection is established despite these barriers, internal processes may be able to stop the infection or delay its progress. One of these is the action of a type of **leukocyte** called a **natural killer cell** (NK). These are activated by proteins called **interferons**, especially produced by cells that are infected with viruses. The specific interferons involved enable the NK cells to recognize those cells that are virus-infected and to destroy them.

The ability to engulf and kill foreign or abnormal cells is an important feature of cells of the innate immune system. Innate immune mechanisms do not

149

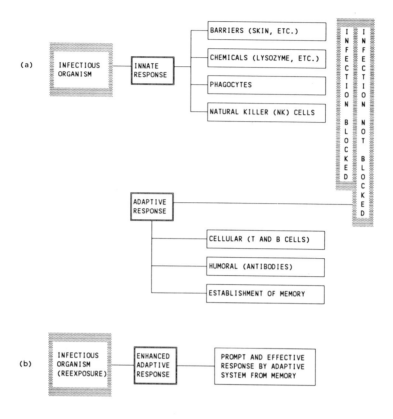

Innate and Adaptive Defense Systems   The innate and adaptive defense systems respond when the body is threatened with infection. This diagram shows the beneficial effects of an enhanced adaptive response that remembers prior contact with an infectious organism.

form a permanent or enhanced resistance to subsequent infections following an initial infection with a particular organism.

ADAPTIVE IMMUNE MECHANISMS

The adaptive immune system establishes a memory for the organism or substance with which it has had contact. A prompt and highly effective response follows a subsequent contact. An adaptive response of the immune system is the formation of antibodies to infectious organisms. The molecular materials, including parts of foreign cell membranes, that stimulate antibody formation are **antigens** (antibody generators).

Sometimes antibodies will react with antigens that are quite similar to the initiating antigen, i.e., **antibody cross-reactions**. This phenomenon allows safe (nondisease-causing) material to produce immune sensitivity to disease-causing

150

(**pathogenic**) organisms. For example, when **cow pox virus** is inoculated into humans, it produces an adaptive immune response that protects against later infection with the serious disease **smallpox**. Similarly, live vaccines are made of viruses (e.g., rabies) that have been adapted to grow in a very different living tissue (e.g., duck embryos). The changed viruses are unable to infect dogs, but they still resemble the initial virus enough to initiate an effective immunity in vaccinated dogs.

T Cells

Some T cells, lymphocytes which have passed through the thymus gland, recognize foreign substances, cells, or organisms by virtue of their own membrane molecules that act as discrete receptors. It also appears that they have the capacity to become genetic subpopulations, each adapted to recognize only one of over a million possible antigens.

Helper T cells react with antigens that have been processed by macrophages; such helper T cells are said to have been **activated**. Some activated T cells enhance the ability of the macrophages to continue engulfing foreign material while others migrate to the spleen and lymph nodes, where they initiate the production of a population of antigen-specific killer T cells.

Killer T cells are able to recognize and destroy cells infected with the specific virus for which the helper T cells have been coded. The mechanism by which NK cells and killer T cells actually kill target cells has been studied. When brought into intimate membrane-to-membrane contact with a target cell, a protein (called **perforin**) is produced that makes holes in the target cell's membrane. Perforation of a cell's membrane results in its death within a few minutes.

Cellular and **humoral** (blood-borne) defenses terminate most infections. However, the matter of terminating the immune activity remains. Suppressor T cells, which matured in the thymus, intervene to stop the immune activities.

Suppressor T cells can prevent helper T cells from triggering the activity of both killer T cells and B cells. There even appears to be a subset of suppressor T cells that monitor the other suppressor T cells and moderate the rate at which the immune process is brought to a halt. After an immune response to an infection is over, a few B and T cells remain and become memory cells for specific antigens. *They initiate such a rapid and effective response that reinfection by that organism may never be possible again.* Suppressor T cells in cancer patients appear to become active too early and inappropriately terminate immune action against cancer cells.

After a slow and uncertain initial period of research, another family of immunologically active proteins and their fragments have been described, the interferons (see sidebar), so named for their ability to interfere with viral multiplication. As many as twenty of these agents are known; the main ones are alpha, beta, and gamma interferons. They are especially significant because they prevent viruses from using a cell's own metabolism to replicate themselves. Certain interferons are involved in antiparasite activity, the killing mechanisms in phagocytes, and destruction of cancer cells.

Interferons

Immune cells and most other cells of an animal's body produce *alpha* and *beta* *interferons*, in response to dead or live viruses and substances secreted by fungi and bacteria. These two interferons prevent viruses from infecting cells.

Gamma interferon exhibits these properties, but it also has other functions; it is produced only by activated T cells while they are engaged in immune responses. Gamma interferon is directed against all microorganisms, including parasites; it appears to activate killing mechanisms in phagocytes.

It has been hoped that the interferons would become effective pharmaceutical agents against infection and cancer—"magic bullets." Except for success in humans against one type of kidney cancer, *hairy-cell leukemia*, and promising results against a few others, the high expectations have not been fulfilled. Certain viral infections may be affected, but further information is still needed to define dosage levels, treatment schedules, and associated treatment.

LYMPHOID ORGANS

The **spleen, lymph nodes**, and **thymus gland** are **lymphoid organs**; they contain stored and transient T cells. The thymus gland is relatively large in an embryo and remains large for a while after birth, although it does not continue to grow as body growth occurs. Puberty marks the beginning of marked reduction in cell mass of the thymus gland. It is responsive to hormones, especially the **adrenocorticoids**. Its reduction in size is especially severe in chronic infections. There is a natural association between thymus gland size reduction during aging and substantial immune changes that accompany aging.

Lymph nodes are stations along the pathways of lymphatic vessels. The immune cells stored in them destroy microorganisms filtered out there. The spleen contains both lymphocytes and macrophages. It filters blood somewhat as the lymph nodes filter the lymph (**interstitial fluid**). Other lymphoid tissues include the **tonsils, adenoids**, and **Peyer's patches** of the intestinal wall.

The thymus also produces a group of polypeptide hormones (**thymosins**), at least one of which is involved in development of the immune competence of T cells. Thymosins act within the thymus and possibly at other sites; injections of some preparations into children with selected immune deficiency conditions have brought about promising results.

THE CONCEPT OF AUTOIMMUNITY

The concept of autoimmunity has brought new understanding to a number of diseases. Yet, it is difficult to reconcile that a function that developed to protect an animal may become destructive under certain circumstances.

In general, autoimmunity increases with age. It is not always clear whether this is because of age-related changes in the immune system or exposure to conditions over time that promote autoimmune processes.

Infectious diseases have been controlled by antibiotics or prevented by immunization. However, diseases caused by the immune system's inappropriate attack on tissues of the self (in contrast to cells from others [nonself]) are now more conspicuous. Until they became better understood and new methods of diagnosing them were developed, they often constituted puzzling conditions.

Some autoimmune diseases are initiated by environmental factors. Injury to tissue may expose proteins or other antigens in such a way that they are not recognizable as self. Penicillin and some other medicines may attach to normal molecules and present an unfamiliar complex to the immune system.

USING IMMUNE PHENOMENA

Development of immunity following certain diseases or inoculation with vaccines is familiar. However, some immune system properties are being exploited for special uses.

Antibodies are so specific that intentional production of them provides tools that recognize special antigens. Many highly specific antibody preparations identify disease organisms in laboratory tests.

Attempts are being made to deliver medical treatment by attachment to specific antibodies for delivery to specific tissue sites. For example, antibodies to unique features of cancer cells can be coupled with a cell **toxin**. Such antibodies seek out only the cancer cells that have the antigen complex they recognize. They then deliver cell-killing toxins to them. Cancer sites that are small, perhaps having spread from a primary cancer site, may be located by antibodies tagged with radioactive atoms.

At the microscopic level, it is then possible to actually identify which cells or intracellular structures take up the tagged antibody; for example, cells with viruses in them can be distinguished.

AGE AND IMMUNITY

ANTIBODIES, IMMUNITY, AND AGE

In dogs, there are natural antibodies to some of their blood group antigens (see the chapter The Blood and Body Fluids). However, aging may be accompanied by a rise in **autoantibodies**—antibodies against the individual's own nucleic acids, mitochondria, stomach cells, thyroglobulin, smooth muscle cells, or even lymphocytes and immunoglobulins themselves. Because some older humans have been shown to have autoantibodies to suppressor T cells, this suggests a mechanism by which immune system regulation in animals is altered with age.

CELL-MEDIATED IMMUNITY AND AGE

Lymphocytes that have been conditioned by the thymus are central to cell-mediated immunity. A reduction in the size of the thymus gland universally accompanies aging, and this would be expected to significantly alter many immune system properties. Although it is probable that immune changes can contribute to some aging, it is just as reasonable that other age-related changes alter the functions of the immune system.

Cell-mediated immunity appears to be less efficient in older animals. Elderly humans do not react as vigorously to the antigens injected into the skin to test for skin reactions. It is not clear whether this is because of a reduced immune memory or alteration of other basic immune responses.

The rejection of foreign tissue grafts is clearly impaired in older animals. In the rejection of tissue grafts, cytotoxic T lymphocytes are the essential, active cells. Their generation, the proliferation of helper T cells, and antigen recognition properties are all needed.

The most conspicuous age-related immune defects seem to be associated with the reduced size of the thymus gland, imbalances in the regulatory T lymphocytes, or shifts toward greater autoimmune activity. Current thinking in the field of immunology holds that changes in immune function may account for some of the increased cancer observed in the aged, and also for some cardiovascular injuries that may initiate cardiovascular disease. Several studies have looked at different measurable immune alterations (e.g., **delayed hypersensitivity**, increased autoantibodies, and reduced suppressor T cell activity) and have correlated them with a shortened life span. However, the altered immunity may have resulted from other factors that resulted in death.

DISEASES OF THE IMMUNE SYSTEM

ANAPHYLAXIS

Anaphylaxis occurs when an antibody reacts with an antigen attached to the membrane of basophils or mast cells. The antigens may be drugs, antibiotics, proteins in serums, venoms, pollens, or complex polysaccharides. The antibody-antigen reaction causes the basophils or mast cells to release a number of biologically active substances, including histamine. The secondary effects are the same symptoms of allergy: respiratory distress caused by spasms of the bronchi, runny nose, or swelling of the vocal cords; gastrointestinal symptoms of vomiting, cramps, or diarrhea; cardiovascular system problems, including low blood pressure and engorgement of blood vessels in the liver and intestines; and skin reactions such as hives. If blood pressure falls sufficiently, the condition of **anaphylactic shock** is said to exist; it is potentially lethal.

Anaphylaxis is not age-related, but it is quite threatening to an older dog. Also, older dogs are more likely to be exposed to some of the antigens, e.g., antibiotics and other drugs. A genetic predisposition for anaphylaxis and allergy exists in some individuals.

IMMUNE SUPPRESSION

As mentioned, suppressor T cells become active in cancer patients and may reduce immune activity of other immune cells. It also appears that some other diseases are associated with temporary immune suppression. Dangerous impairment of the immune system accompanies severe malnutrition. However, some caloric restriction delays aging of the immune system (see the chapter Nutrition and Metabolism). Changes that accompany thymus involution are discussed above.

Drugs that are used following organ transplants are meant to cause immune suppression. Many of those used to suppress cancer cell growth similarly affect immune function. Other medicines have immunosuppressive side effects; some seriously damage the bone marrow, the original source of immune cells.

AUTOIMMUNE DISEASES OF THE MUSCULOSKELETAL SYSTEM

Canine rheumatoid arthritis results when tissues of the joints become injured by an immune attack. It resembles rheumatoid arthritis in humans, but it seems to have characteristics unique to the dog. It is believed that some aspects of this disease in humans may be genetic and this may be true in dogs. It is typical in small and Toy breeds and in young or middle-aged dogs, but it is seen in larger and older animals. Rheumatoid arthritis is quite different from osteoarthritis, which is notably age-related (see the chapter The Skeleton and Skeletal Muscles).

The joints of dogs in which symptoms first appear are in the feet, but symptoms may later involve larger joints. Pain, stiff movement, and swelling of tissue near the inflamed joints are characteristic. Joint deformity is common in this destructive process.

Canine rheumatoid arthritis cannot be cured at the present time. Occasionally, spontaneous remission may occur; remission following treatment with immunosuppressive drugs also has been observed. At first, corticosteroids may relieve symptoms, but continued use may contribute to increased joint damage.

Your veterinarian can test for a blood protein called **rheumatoid factor** (RF). Rheumatoid factor is commonly, but not always, present and is also found in other diseases. It is not an easily diagnosed disease, considering how many inflammatory joint conditions may be associated with diseases. Only your veterinarian can place your dog on the most acceptable medication.

Nonerosive polyarthritis is an inflammatory condition of various joints that often develops following infectious diseases. The mechanism that initiates the arthritic changes is not fully understood, but immune complexes may be involved. It has sometimes been incorrectly diagnosed as a neurological condition because of an affected dog's inability to walk or its paralyzed appearance. Your veterinarian will differentiate this condition from other diseases with similar features. Attention to the associated infection is the primary treatment. Corticosteroids are sometimes used along with other measures.

In **myasthenia gravis**, voluntary muscles become weak because an immune attack damages the receptors for the neurotransmitter **acetylcholine**. This prevents nerve impulses from reaching a muscle's cells (see the chapters The Excitable Tissues and The Skeleton and Skeletal Muscles). It is a condition found in dogs, cats, and humans; and it is not predominant in the aged. Symptoms can be treated, but the disease is not yet curable. It is a grave disease when the muscles of the swallowing reflex and the respiratory system become involved.

Immune damage to the myelin sheaths of neurons appears to occur in a form of **distemper encephalitis**. Movement difficulties and other muscular symptoms may accompany the resultant alteration in nerve conduction.

Polymyositis is an inflammation of the skeletal muscles of the body. It may be possible to feel the swollen and contracted muscles (see the chapter The Skeleton and Skeletal Muscles). After time, some muscles may atrophy. Muscles throughout the body are susceptible, and the symptoms and seriousness of the condition relate to which ones are involved. The autoantibody involved in polymyositis appears to be against some part of the muscle cell nucleus.

Your veterinarian must make sure that other conditions such as polyarthritis, meningitis, or spinal cord injuries are not mistaken for polymyositis. For diagnosis, microscopic muscle samples may be needed, along with electrical recording of the muscles (**electromyograph**). Also, several muscle enzymes are released into the blood and may be measured. If the dog is free of infection, corticosteroids may be helpful.

AUTOIMMUNITY AND THE BLOOD AND LYMPHATIC SYSTEM

Autoimmune hemolytic anemia (AIHA) is somewhat common in the dog. It is caused by antibodies against the red blood cells that make them rupture. AIHA rapidly progresses and is characterized by depression, weakness, and the pale mucous membranes seen in anemias. When it becomes severe, fainting, breathing difficulty, fast heart rate, and other symptoms appear. The hemoglobin released from destroyed red blood cells may damage the kidneys. Other circumstances that may burden the kidneys must be avoided at this time.

Blood transfusions may be needed if the anemia is very severe. Certain corticosteroids are useful in carefully monitored treatment. This is a serious disease; its outcome is varied, depending on a number of factors that include severity and any underlying diseases.

Immune-mediated thrombocytopenia (IMT) is a condition in which blood platelets are destroyed by antibodies that have developed against them. As is the case of low platelet counts from any cause, an increased tendency to bleed is seen. Small hemorrhages may be visible in the mouth. Accompanying symptoms may include fever, anemia, enlarged lymph nodes, and enlarged liver and spleen.

Immune-mediated thrombocytopenia is difficult to diagnose because it may resemble other conditions. Bone marrow samples are useful because it is possible to examine the health of the bone marrow cells from which platelets come. The outcome of treatment is variable; prognosis and treatment resemble that for AIHA.

AUTOIMMUNE DISEASES OF THE ENDOCRINE SYSTEM

Hypothyroidism (see the chapter The Endocrine System), a common problem in dogs, may often have an immune cause. **Autoimmune thyroiditis** in the dog resembles Hashimoto's disease in humans. Antibodies to **thyroglobulin** (a storage form of thyroid hormone) are found in the blood.

In humans, **Type I diabetes mellitus** begins primarily in the young (see the chapter The Endocrine System). Antibodies to insulin, to insulin receptors on cells, or to the pancreatic cells that produce insulin have been demonstrated. In dogs that are dependent on insulin injections, some of these undesired immune reactions appear to be present. Obviously, more research will help improve veterinary care in young and older dogs with insulin-dependent diabetes.

WIDESPREAD AUTOIMMUNE DISEASES

Amyloidosis may not be a good term for a disease. It actually describes those conditions in which deposits of amyloid are found in any of the body's tissues. These deposits include fragments of antibody molecules, and damage to tissues seems to involve the injury from an immune attack. Much more research is needed to provide knowledge in this area.

In addition to the central nervous system, amyloid deposits have been reported in the kidneys, spleen, liver, and adrenal glands. In dogs, the presence of amyloid appears to be secondary to various infectious diseases, including bone infection (**osteomyelitis**) and **tuberculosis**. Various cancers may coexist. When liver disease is associated with amyloid deposits, an enlarged liver, abnormal liver function tests, and bile duct obstruction may be found. Deposits of amyloid are found in some cases of **glomerulonephritis** (inflammation of the glomeruli of the kidney), which is a condition also seen in **systemic lupus erythematosus** (SLE). The damage to the glomeruli permits protein, especially albumin, to be lost into the urine, causing the many effects of low blood protein (see the chapters The Cardiovascular System and The Blood and Body Fluids).

Systemic lupus erythematosus is a very serious disease, although its cause is not clear. Genetic, hormonal, and viral influences have been cited. It is known that suppressor T cell function is altered. DNA of cells and other tissue components are damaged by immune attack. Therefore, many organs are injured. The condition may vary between different dogs because symptoms depend on the pattern of organs involved.

Arthritic symptoms, protein excretion into the urine, skin inflammation, anemia, low white blood cell counts, and reduced blood platelets may all accompany SLE. One of the very serious lesions is degeneration in the blood vessel lining. Death from SLE is commonly from kidney failure.

Corticosteroids and immunosuppressive drugs have been used to treat SLE. Cure is not possible at this time, but some cases will do well for a few years under treatment.

AUTOIMMUNE DISEASES OF THE SKIN

The skin diseases that are related to an autoimmune reaction resemble many other skin diseases.

Pemphigus foliaceus is the most common autoimmune skin disease in dogs. The intercellular cement substance is injured by an autoimmune antibody against it. The symptoms gradually appear; the area around the eyes, ears, and the nose are primarily affected. These areas show hair loss, reddening, pustules, and scab formation. Occasionally, other areas of the body are involved.

Pemphigus erythematosus is similar to pemphigus foliaceus, developing gradually, and appearing in the same primary areas. Skin areas involved lose their pigment, and the lesions may be made worse by exposure to sunlight.

Pemphigus vulgaris is usually not as mild as the above; its onset is acute and the dog is severely ill. Ulcerations and erosions may be found also in the oral mucosa and the nail beds.

In the case of **bullous pemphigoid**, the autoantibody is directed toward an antigen in the basement membrane where epidermis joins the dermis. The lesions bring about significant loss of the epidermal layer in dogs. Lesions in the acute form include reddening and ulcer formation of the oral mucosa. In the acute form, dogs may have fever and general symptoms of illness. On the other hand, chronically affected animals may have generalized lesions, but their overall condition is more benign. Collies and Doberman Pinschers seem especially susceptible to bullous pemphigoid.

Discoid lupus erythematosus resembles SLE in several respects. However, it is not a systemic disease, and it is relatively benign.

158

In both of the lupus diseases, changes in the skin are similar. Skin lesions show reddening, loss of pigment, and scarring. The nose, ears, and head are affected in SLE and discoid lupus erythematosus. The skin lesions in both diseases are sensitive to sunlight.

ALTERING THE IMMUNE SYSTEM

As the complex role of the immune system becomes more evident, especially the possibility that its function is related to life span, ways to control immune functions are sought. Some books that are intended as human nutrition guides suggest ways to use diet to manipulate the immune system; they are popular and probably quite misleading. Yet the relationships between the immune system and the endocrine system, as well as the nervous system, are fruitful areas for careful future research.

Dietary restriction does extend life span in laboratory animals (see the chapter Nutrition and Metabolism). In diet-restricted animals, the thymus gland does not undergo reduction in size as early, and many immune functions are sustained for a longer time.

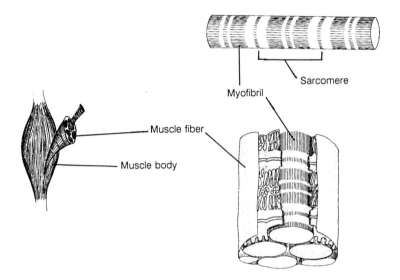

Sarcomere

Myofibril

Muscle fiber

Muscle body

Skeletal Muscle   A skeletal muscle is composed of bundles of muscle groups. A muscle fiber is the equivalent of a cell, but is actually several cells combined into one functional unit. The muscle fiber is composed of a number of strands called *myofibrils*, each of which is a series of units called *sarcomeres*—the parts of the muscle that shorten to cause contraction.

14

The Skeleton and Skeletal Muscles: Movement and Posture

***

$\mathbf{M}$USCLE AND BONE are dissimilar in many respects. Each has its own unique metabolism, and the anatomy of bone and muscle could not be more different. Yet, the two work together, each dependent on the other. The role of bone and muscle in locomotion is obvious. However, the importance of the two in positioning or anchoring much of the body in order to support movement of other parts is often overlooked.

Both of these tissues are important reservoirs of metabolic substances. Muscle is a major source of amino acids when dietary protein is low, and muscle mass is reduced in aged animals. Bone is not only composed of calcium compounds, the calcium, phosphorus, and magnesium in it are also available to other parts of the body when the supply is low.

MUSCLE STRUCTURE AND CONTRACTION

The electrical properties of muscle are examined in the chapter The Excitable Tissues. Muscle resembles nervous tissue in this respect. The role of proteins in the contraction of muscle is presented (see accompanying sidebar), and this is a good example of the relationship between composition and function. **Skeletal muscle**, **cardiac muscle**, and **smooth muscle** use the same reactant

161

Muscle Contraction

Several proteins found within each *sarcomere* interact to bring about contraction. The *thin filaments* are parallel chains of many small, globular protein molecules known as *actin*. *Thick filaments* consist of large, long protein molecules (*myosin*), also arranged in a parallel fashion. A particular feature of the bundled myosin molecules is that they have terminal structures that have been described as knobs or heads, structures that stick out conspicuously from the bundle. These knobs form transient bonds (*bridges*) with the actin molecules during muscle contraction.

Myosin knobs are ordinarily prevented from forming bridges because the reactive sites on the actin molecules are covered by molecules of another protein, *tropomyosin*. When calcium ions are released into the *myofibril*, they bring about a shifting of the position of tropomyosin so that the knobs of myosin can form a cross-bridge with actin molecules. The cross-bridging triggers the release of high energy from molecules of ATP. This release of high energy results in intramolecular forces that cause the knobs to change position. The effect of this attachment, followed by repeated repositioning of the myosin knobs, is to pull myosin along the length of the actin chains. Because this event is a rapid and recurrent one, and is occurring at both ends of the myosin, the actin filaments from both ends of the sarcomere are drawn toward the center and cause each sarcomere to shorten. This resembles the action of a ratchet and is called the "sliding filament theory of contraction." Although calcium is the mediator of this remarkable phenomenon, nerve impulses initiate the pulses of calcium release.

molecules for contraction. However, cells from each kind of muscle differ in certain ways. The following discussion is about skeletal muscle.

A fibrous **connective tissue** sheath surrounds a muscle. It is the same material as the **tendons** that attach muscles to the skeleton. Smaller bundles, muscle **fasciculi**, further organize muscle. These in turn are each composed of a number of **muscle fibers**, which are modified muscle cells. Finally, each muscle fiber is made up of several long units known as **myofibrils** that are the primary functional parts of the muscle.

The electron microscope, with its ability to magnify thousands of times, has provided detailed knowledge of the structure of myofibrils.

MUSCLE AND AGING

Because skeletal muscle fibers (cells) cannot reproduce, they are not replaced when lost because of injury or disease. This loss could explain the characteristic reduction in strength and muscle mass during aging. Lack of use also results in muscle wasting. Yet, muscle fibers given appropriate exercise can increase in size, partly compensating for the loss of fibers.

However, many other factors must be considered if loss of strength and muscle mass is observed. The brain itself may fail to initiate muscle contraction, especially if restricted blood flow in the brain impairs its function. Because nerve pathways consist of a series of neurons with chemical connections between them, errors in an appropriate chemical **neurotransmitter** (see the chapter The Excitable Tissues) can cause some of these effects (e.g., myasthenia gravis).

All excitable tissue depends upon a suitable electrolyte/water balance. Thus, imbalance of the concentrations of sodium, calcium, or potassium can have profound effects. Muscle tissue depends on a suitable local pH (acid/base balance), which is maintained by effective lung and kidney function. Adequate protein intake, digestion, and metabolism are required for the synthesis of muscle proteins. The presence of adequate amounts of the energy-releasing **adenosine triphosphate** (ATP) is also a function of suitable nutrition and metabolism.

The paragraph above does not explain all considerations of factors related to muscle function. It does, however, make the point that simplistic answers are not likely to be appropriate when explaining the observations of aging phenomena.

DISEASES OF MUSCLE

Diseases of muscles are called **myopathies**, some of which are referred to as a **myositis** (inflammation of muscle). Muscles may be injured by physical trauma, infection, loss of blood circulation, excessive use, inappropriate nutrition, and various toxins. Naturally, locomotion and posture are affected whenever muscles fail to perform properly. Eye movement, eating and drinking, and respiration are also body functions that may be compromised when muscles

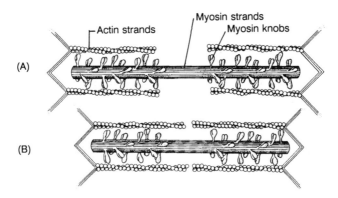

Actin-Myosin Reaction This illustrates how the strands of the thick filaments (myosin) react with the thin filaments (actin) to shorten a sarcomere. In (A), the sarcomere is in a resting state; (B) shows the ends of the sarcomere pulled inward by the progressive interaction between the two types of filaments. The accompanying sidebar provides more details of the reaction.

malfunction. Skeletal muscle is dependent on the receipt of motor nerve impulses, which requires proper neuromuscular transmitter metabolism (e.g., **acetylcholine** metabolism).

Primarily identified in German Shepherd Dogs, **eosinophilic myositis** has a rapid onset and most often affects the muscles needed for chewing. It is a relapsing disease, returning within weeks or months. It may become worse with subsequent attacks. At rest, the mouth is held partially open, and eating elicits considerable pain. It is diagnosed by its breed preference, symptoms, and a high **eosinophil** count in the blood (**eosinophilia**). Sometimes a muscle biopsy (sample) is examined. Corticosteroids may provide some relief, but an effective treatment is not known.

Myasthenia gravis may be congenital or acquired. Only the acquired type is likely to be seen in older dogs. This form is characterized by an autoimmune attack (see the chapter The Protective Role of the Immune System) against the muscle membrane receptors for the neurotransmitter acetylcholine (see the chapter The Excitable Tissues). Thus, impulses via nerves to muscle cells are not effective. In addition to general weakness, changes in the dog's bark and swallowing difficulties may indicate this disease. Relapses and remissions of the condition may occur, and medical treatment is helpful.

Idiopathic polymyositis is the term used to describe a fairly common muscle disease in dogs, mostly in adults of large breeds. The usual muscle weakness, gait changes, and muscle loss are seen, as in many muscle diseases, but the cause of this particular condition is not known (i.e., it is idiopathic). Your veterinarian may need a muscle biopsy to confirm a diagnosis. Prompt use of corticosteroids is often effective, especially in acute cases. If the condition is chronic and progressive, treatment may have little effect.

A **progressive myopathy** occasionally afflicts dogs, and it is seen primarily in older dogs. It resembles **muscular dystrophy** (MS) in humans. It is probably inherited in some cases; that certainly is the case in other animals that have been studied. As in the human disease, the course of the disease in dogs may vary. Weakness and alterations in gait accompany the loss of muscle mass. Blood tests can help your veterinarian establish a diagnosis. Effective treatment is not now available, and the prognosis is poor for dogs with this progressive disease.

BONE STRUCTURE AND METABOLISM

The shapes of bones reflect well-known physical functions. However, bone is also an important reservoir of calcium, phosphorus, and magnesium. Because of this, bone is involved in several types of metabolism. Important information on calcium metabolism is in the chapter Nutrition and Metabolism.

A typical bone consists of a spongy portion surrounded by more compact bone. Healthy spongy bone is quite strong because of the arrangement of bony plates that comprise it. It is abundant near the ends of supporting bones. The shaft of a long bone is a rigid tube; a **medullary cavity** runs down its center, which is filled with a collection of fat and **bone marrow** cells (see the chapter The Blood and Body Fluids).

At a microscopic level, bone cells (**osteocytes**) are found in chambers within bone structure. However, they are not isolated from one another because they send out small cellular extensions providing communication between them. Small blood vessels follow canals in the bone mass to provide nutrients and waste disposal and to permit exposure to appropriate hormones and vitamins.

Bone cells known as **osteoblasts** form bone by removing calcium and phosphate from the blood to form crystals of **hydroxyapatite**. This is added to the cartilage that provides shape to bones. **Osteoclasts** are cells that erode bone by breaking down the hydroxyapatite, returning the chemical elements to the blood. Both of these cells function simultaneously so that bone is a result of a balanced combination of their activities.

The chapter The Endocrine System describes the functions of hormones such as **parathyroid hormone, calcitonin, active vitamin D, growth hormone, thyroid hormone**, and sex hormones **testosterone** and **estrogen** (see also the chapter The Reproductive System). All of these have been found to have significant influences on bone physiology. A deficiency of vitamin D results in poor bone formation, a condition known as **rickets** in immature animals. A vitamin D deficiency in adults allows a net calcium loss, and the condition called **osteomalacia** develops. Excess absorption of calcium without appropriate phosphorus and magnesium actually decreases proper bone metabolism and may also contribute to other conditions such as arthritis and kidney stones.

THE SKELETON AND AGING

Loss of bone tissue takes place as aging occurs. Although this loss appears to be universal, the rate at which it is lost varies from dog to dog; genetic factors, nutrition, and physical conditioning all play roles. However, the activity of osteoblasts, which produce bone and contribute to its mineralization, decreases considerably with age. Because collagen synthesis is needed for formation of bone, it is reasonable to believe that it is deficient in bone, as it is in skin and other tissues of older animals.

In ways not yet understood, physical activity provides a stimulus for bone formation. The reduced activity of older dogs may contribute to reduction in bone mineralization.

The bone marrow space increases as bone mass decreases. However, fat in the marrow space increases, and there is actually a reduction in functional bone marrow cells (see the chapter The Blood and Body Fluids).

At least in humans, calcium absorption in the intestine is reduced; an inadequate source of vitamin D will add to this problem. Common age-related changes in endocrine function may bring about changes in bone metabolism, particularly corticosteroid secretion, thyroid hormone production, or parathyroid gland function.

BONE AND JOINT DISEASES

The prevalence of **secondary osteoporosis** (loss of bone and its density) increases in older dogs, but it is less conspicuous than in humans, where it is considered a primary condition (see the chapter Nutrition and Metabolism). Serious bone weakness occurs, bone fractures increase, and an altered posture may develop.

Fundamentally, osteoporosis may result from inadequate intake or absorption of calcium, but an inadequate amount of phosphorus or magnesium may be at fault. Abnormal processing of calcium by bone-synthesizing cells or bone-eroding cells, excessive excretion of calcium relative to intake, and other factors are possible factors affecting bone density.

Osteitis is the term that applies to inflammation of bone; inflammation of the bone marrow is called **osteomyelitis**. Bacterial infection is usually the cause. Most of the cases are infections secondary to physical injury (blows or bite wounds) or orthopedic surgery. Disease of dental support tissues also may be a source of osteitis. Pain that is localized to an area of bone, swelling, and fever related to the bacterial infection are among the symptoms. Although aggressive, long-term treatment of the infection is important, success is not assured. Amputation or surgical removal of bone is sometimes required.

Bone tissue is subject to cancer; by far, the most common is **osteosarcoma**. This cancer is seen in dogs over a wide range of age, but eight years old is the most common age reported. Boxers, Collies, German Shepherds, Great Danes, Irish Setters, and Saint Bernards appear more predisposed than other breeds. The symptoms of lameness and local swelling have a rapid onset. This cancer quite frequently metastasizes to the lungs. An X-ray will assist your veterinarian in diagnosing osteosarcoma. However, there are few ways to treat this rapidly developing tumor. Although many cancer-suppressing drugs are available, none provide much promise at present. Amputation of an affected limb may provide brief relief of pain, but it does not seem to prolong life.

Chondrosarcoma (a cancer of cartilage cells) is a much less common cancer. It appears in slightly younger dogs, on average, than osteosarcoma. This cancer tends to originate in the nasal area, ribs, or pelvic bone structure. The symptoms are determined by the location of the lesions. If these tumors can be completely removed surgically, prognosis is good. Tumors that are primary to other sites may spread to the bone. Also, tumors of bone, benign or malignant, may cause secondary effects; e.g., pressure on blood vessels supplying bone may cause bone cell death from lack of sufficient blood flow.

Hypertrophic osteoarthropathy occurs primarily in older dogs. It is characterized by growths along the surface of various bones. Lameness, pain, and swelling are common symptoms. Large tumors or growths in the chest area are present in a great number of dogs with hypertrophic osteoarthropathy, but it is not known what causes the bone membrane to initiate these growths on bone surfaces. X-ray images help diagnose the condition by providing images of both the chest and bone surfaces. The only treatment that appears useful is to remove the chest masses, if possible. If malignant growths are present, death from the cancer is likely.

Osteoarthritis is the most common joint disease in dogs; it is very age-related, being most common in dogs ten years old or older. Unlike rheumatoid arthritis (see the chapter The Protective Role of the Immune System), osteoarthritis is not always accompanied by pain. The weight-bearing joints are the ones most affected.

This is a degenerative disease that may have injury, infection of joints, and genetic malformation as factors; the causes of all cases are not understood. Any joint is susceptible, but the ones that bear weight are most often involved. In dogs, **canine hip dysplasia** leads to osteoarthritis, but any condition that makes a joint unstable can do the same. Dogs with osteoarthritis may have pain in affected joints; they may limp and suppress their activity. Because the pain and deterioration is worsened by excessive exercise, care should be taken to encourage only enough regular exercise to help maintain mobility. Your veterinarian can distinguish this from other conditions by using X-ray examination of the joints and other signs. Appropriate exercise such as walking and swimming, effective rest, weight reduction in fat dogs, and anti-inflammatory drugs such as aspirin and corticosteroids are primary ways of treating the condition.

Older dogs may have a blood-borne bacterial infection (a **septicemia**) that develops following many tissue infections, especially of the urinary tract, skin, mouth, and respiratory system. The infectious organisms reach skeletal joints by way of the blood and cause arthritic conditions, perhaps more frequently in larger dogs. Pain and swelling may occur, and your veterinarian will use an awareness of the primary infection, blood tests, and X-ray examination of affected joints for diagnosis. Prompt treatment of the primary infection is required in order to stop the injury to joints and to prevent further complications such as osteomyelitis.

Canine hip dysplasia (CHD) is a genetically predisposed disease that becomes troublesome as affected dogs become older. It is characterized by hip joints in which the head of the **femur** (long bone of the leg) does not fit properly into the hip socket (**acetabulum**). Too great a freedom of movement of this joint leads to inflammation and progressive damage. It is now known that other joints may be similarly involved. Large breeds have more CHD than smaller ones, but males and females are equally affected. Young dogs do not show symptoms. Diagnosis is by the use of carefully prepared special X-ray examinations that are interpreted by specialists familiar with the condition.

Studies of genetic factors show that more than one gene is probably involved; thus, the condition is difficult to predict. Although environmental factors play a part, there is no question that dogs with CHD have more offspring with the condition than dogs showing no signs of it. The best current hope of reducing or eradicating the disease is selective breeding.

Once CHD has developed, gentle exercise is beneficial; excessive exercise is damaging. Aspirin and other medications control some pain, but dietary supplements are not useful. While nothing is known that will arrest the disease, an accelerated growth rate in puppies seems to promote earlier development of CHD.

Intervertebral disk disease is often classified as a neurological disease because of the neurological symptoms that follow pressure on the spinal cord (see the chapter The Central Nervous System). It is, however, a joint condition to the extent that it involves extrusion of the material that separates the vertebrae from each other into the space containing the spinal cord and spinal nerves. All breeds may have the condition, but dogs such as the Beagle, Cocker Spaniel, Dachshund, Pekingese, Poodle, Shih Tzu, and Welsh Corgi, often long-bodied, are most commonly effected. Symptoms are related to the area of the spinal column and the number of intervertebral disks involved. Pain, leg paralysis, urinary incontinence, and, in some cases, respiratory paralysis are among the symptoms of intervertebral disk disease. X-ray examination helps a veterinarian diagnose and evaluate the extent of spinal cord damage. The usual painkillers and anti-inflammatory drugs may be used in mild or early cases. However, surgery is likely to be your veterinarian's choice, and the long recovery period and nursing care will require dedication.

Spondylosis deformans (**ankylosing spondylitis**) is also a degenerative condition of old dogs involving the vertebrae, especially in the lumbar area. It is usually without pain until pressure develops on nerve roots in the affected area. This condition is more common in large, active breeds of dogs.

Patellar luxation (dislocation of the kneecap) found often in Toy and miniature breeds of dogs, is found in all sizes of dogs. It appears to have an inherited component, but is often seen in older dogs as a result of trauma to an already disordered patellar support structure. When seen in larger dogs, it occurs in the early months of life in those breeds commonly affected by hip dysplasia. Surgery is the main form of treatment; however, it is successful in a limited number of cases.

Ligaments (**anterior cruciate** or **posterior cruciate**) of the **stifle** and **patella** are often affected by a progressive degeneration that continues into a dog's later years. Obesity makes the problem more severe. Rupture of the ligament, particularly the anterior cruciate ligament, can occur in older dogs as they run or jump; the dog will at first carry the affected leg off the ground and only gradually try to use it again. The unstable joint may lead to joint disease and damage to other associated tissue. These possibilities must by taken into account in evaluating the condition. Some dogs, especially smaller ones, often improve without surgery. However, your veterinarian will advise you of proper treatment. Surgical repair is quite successful.

15

The Skin:
Temperature Control
and Body Defense

STRUCTURE AND PHYSIOLOGY OF SKIN

The dog's skin is exposed to many environmental hazards. Although the lungs come into contact with an enormous volume of air, parts of the skin are subjected to chemically active ultraviolet light, physical trauma, and deleterious airborne substances. The hair coat participates in protection of the surface; its amount varies with genetic differences and with the seasonal length of days.

The skin is one of the body's largest and most extensive organ systems. The health and well-being of the skin and its appendages (toenails, hair) provide an opportunity to study several different aspects of aging, such as cross-linking in collagen or the rate of healing following injury. *Skin can constitute nearly one-quarter of a dog's body weight, depending on the size and age of the dog.*

Disorders of the skin are major causes for visits of dogs to a veterinarian. Some skin diseases are serious and life-threatening while others are primarily uncomfortable or disfiguring. At times, alterations in cells or structure of the skin are primary causes of skin disease. However, the skin's condition often serves as a diagnostic window to disease in other parts of the body.

The skin's physiological roles include temperature control, water balance, excretory activity, hormone activation (vitamin D), protective functions (barrier and immunological), and sensory input. The **mammary glands** (breasts) are modified skin glands. Fat storage involves skin to a great degree. In many animals, including dogs, scent glands reside in the skin and can transmit signals to other individuals. The skin also has abundant **lymph** capillaries to help drain sites of infection toward **lymph nodes**. The hair and toenails are skin appendages.

Epidermal Layers—Cells and Organization

The **epidermis** is the outermost layer of skin. It is a constantly renewing layer and the surface cells are essentially dead cells. The effect of ultraviolet (UV) light from the sun, which is damaging to many molecules, is moderated by the fact that this layer is constantly shed and replaced with undamaged cells. The epidermis contains three types of cells: **keratinocytes**, **melanocytes**, and **Langerhans cells**. The last, *not to be confused with the islets of Langerhans of the pancreas*, are the least abundant; they appear to function in **antigen** recognition and processing, thus serving an immunological role.

The **dermis**, the layer below the epidermis, exerts a continuous influence

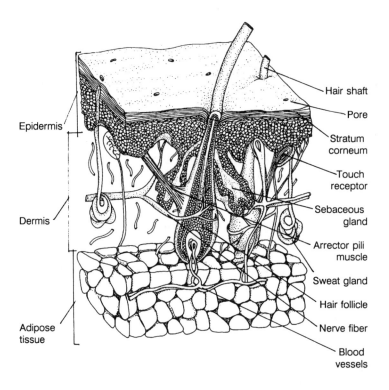

Anatomy of Mammalian Skin This illustrates a composite of typical features of skin and its associated elements. See the text for discussion of many of the parts.

by producing a growth-stimulating substance. Another **epidermal growth factor** has been extracted from the salivary gland. Cell division in the epidermis is stimulated by vitamin A, and it is inhibited by certain corticosteroids and by adrenaline, which complexes with the growth factors.

The melanocytes are pigment-forming cells that are responsible for skin color. These cells synthesize the pigment **melanin**, which is part of cells carrying color. Melanocyte activity is more evident in some areas such as about the nipples, the anus, the genital area, and, sometimes, the eyes; it is associated with **hair follicles** and provides the pigment for hair color. Genetic variants of melanin are evident in various hair colors.

The keratinocytes are the most abundant of all epidermal cells. During embryonic life, some of these cells penetrate lower levels of the skin and give rise to hair follicles and skin glands. These cells produce fibrous proteins known as **keratins**, which are quite stable.

The outermost keratinocytes (the horny layer) are in a position to serve a barrier function. They are relatively water-resistant by virtue of the oily secretions of the skin's **sebaceous glands**. Baths with soap interfere with their water-shedding property and remove surface cells somewhat sooner than they would have been shed. It is not clear whether this exposes cells that are more sensitive to injury from environmental influences. Serious errors in the process of forming keratin are associated with some genetic disorders of fat metabolism.

The Dermis—The Second Skin Layer

The dermis is rich in connective tissue, varying considerably from one area to another. **Fibroblasts** are the principal cells in the dermis, and their products, especially **collagen** and **elastin**, are abundant. Most of the dry weight of the dermis is collagen, several subtypes being present. The fibers of collagen are formed into a diamond-shaped network. Stretching the skin aligns the fibers along the tension lines. This enables restoration of the skin to its original orientation, with the help of elastin fibers. **Fibronectin** is a glycoprotein found at the dermis-epidermis junction, and it is associated with hairs, blood vessels, and nerves. It appears to serve as a binding agent, including the binding of cells to collagen. Several substances make up an amorphous **ground substance** in which the cells and fibers of the dermis are embedded. This is a gel-like matrix containing blood vessels, nerves, lymphatic channels, gland ducts, and hair follicles.

Skin Glands

Sweat glands are widely distributed in humans, but are found only on the foot pads in dogs. As mentioned in the chapter The Respiratory System, dogs use evaporation of water from the nasal passages as a major means of cooling. Temperature control also relies on skin blood flow and the coat with its ability to trap air.

Sebaceous glands develop from and are associated with hair follicles. Their product is a fatty material. It lubricates the hair follicle and coats hair and skin surfaces, waterproofing them and providing a mild bactericidal and fungistatic action. Activity of sebaceous glands is quite sensitive to male sex hormone levels. This sensitivity explains why they become active after puberty and sometimes regress in older individuals.

Hair and Toenails—Growth and Composition

Hair is an insoluble material containing proteins and produced in hair follicles by a process that alters cells, which are then pressed into a cylindrical shape as they leave the follicle. Thus, the shaft of a hair is specially modified epidermal cells. Melanin and related molecules are contributed by associated melanocytes, which become less numerous with age, accounting for the loss of pigment in hair, as in graying or whitening of hair.

Hair follicles vary in activity according to the length of daylight. Thus, they may alternate between an active and inactive state. A special phase also occurs at least once a year when molting or shedding takes place, usually in late spring or fall. Other influences that increase hair growth include increased thyroid hormone and decreased adrenal gland and sex hormones. On the other hand, excess corticosteroids and estrogens inhibit hair growth. Spayed females have no ovaries to produce estrogens; their coats are likely to be smooth and soft. An imbalance in diet may also affect hair and coat quality.

Toenails are more primitive than hair, the latter being present only in mammals. Feathers, scales, etc., are characteristic of lower animals; some form of toenails are found far down the evolutionary scale. The **nail bed**, on which the nail rests, has epidermal and dermal layers. At its rear, the epidermal layer serves as a site from which the nail grows, which is similar to the production of hairs. Here, cells are modified and added to the base of the nail to provide its growth. In the dog, a rich blood vessel and nerve supply runs down part of the nail shaft.

Blood Supply to Skin

The skin has a blood supply in excess of its own circulatory needs. Hair follicles and sebaceous glands are richly supplied with capillary beds. There is an arterial network just beneath the dermis that sends blood vessel branches into tissue above it. Extensive connections exist between smaller arteries and veins; these provide a means of shunting blood away from the skin. When these shunts are constricted, blood is forced to flow through vessels near the skin surface. This provides a mechanism for retaining body heat or losing it more readily. The pattern of blood flow is controlled by local reflexes and by the **hypothalamus**, which monitors body temperature. In dogs, a well-developed hair coat and a great ability to regulate blood flow in the skin allows them to tolerate environmental temperatures much lower than tolerated by humans.

Nerves of the Skin

Motor nerves go to skin glands and **arrector pili** muscles along the hair follicles. These small muscles are able to make hair stand erect and cause the puckering of the skin known as "goose bumps."

The skin is well recognized as a significant site of sensory input. Temperature receptors help regulate a number of temperature control reflexes such as shivering, modification of metabolic rate, secretion by the nasal water gland, and sweating. Tactile stimulation, including distortion of hair position, initiates conscious responses such as scratching an itch, licking a mildly painful area, etc. **Prostaglandins, histamine**, and a number of chemicals may participate in stimulation reactions of the skin. Also, the skin contains specific sensory receptors for pain, heat, and cold.

Subcutaneous Fat

Beneath the two layers of skin is a layer of fat, the **subcutaneous fat**. It varies from one area to another in familiar patterns, and it varies in total amount from one animal to another. It is an excellent thermal insulator, and it is a natural store of potential energy for metabolism. If present in excess, it may provide too much insulation for hot environments.

AGING AND THE SKIN

Skin wrinkles, changes in skin pigmentation, hair loss, and graying are signs of aging. It is especially difficult to separate age-related diseases of the skin from changes in skin caused by progressive age alone. However, changes in skin resulting from changes in the amount and arrangement of collagen fibers may reflect similar alterations in collagen metabolism known to take place in diseased tissue elsewhere.

Appearance of Aging Skin

One age-related change in skin appearance is associated with the loss of subcutaneous fat in some areas, although total body fat may be increased. The fat beneath the dermis models the skin above it into features of the face, etc. This is modified by sagging and deep folds. In addition, changes in collagen and elastin allow skin to sag, and when stretched, it returns to its original position more slowly than young skin.

Body Temperature Control and Aging

Fat loss is only a part of a diminished ability to retain heat in old dogs. The small blood vessels of the skin are less abundant and less well organized in the elderly, associated in part with the reduction in dermal (*not* epidermal) thickness. Skin that has been injured by chronic sun exposure has a great reduction in its microvasculature. The capillary beds around hair follicles and skin glands are reduced, contributing to reduced skin gland function and hair growth observed in the aged.

In a cold environment, older individuals' blood vessels may fail to constrict and they may not shiver as readily so that the core body temperature falls. This indicates possible combinations of lowered sensory input to the hypothalamus, inadequate hypothalamic function, and deficient motor responses in the skin's microvascular system and skeletal muscles. In extreme cold, lessening of pain perception may cause the elderly to ignore proper protection, such as relocation to warmer places.

Exposure to high temperatures is also not well tolerated by the elderly. Heat stroke is easily experienced, especially if the nasal cooling mechanism is inefficient and sufficient skin blood flow cannot be accomplished.

Impaired Wound Healing

In order to assure good wound healing in the elderly dog, longer wound healing periods are needed, special attention should be paid to surgical technique, and extended nursing care must be provided. Many modern studies have confirmed the delayed wound repair in older animals when strength of the wound, rate of collagen deposition, regeneration of the skin above blisters, or the incorporation of radioactively tagged substrates into new tissue are measured.

The Skin and Immunity

A relatively new area of study is the effect of the skin on immune phenomena. Cellular and humoral immunity are both reduced in the elderly. Some serious autoimmune disorders are characteristic of older animals (see the chapter The Protective Role of the Immune System). The new discipline of **photoimmunology** has demonstrated that excessive exposure to the sun has immunological consequences throughout the body by inducing **suppressor T cells**. This impairs the **immune surveillance system**, allowing cancer to be initiated and persist.

Hair Graying and Slow Growth

Hair graying, especially about the muzzle, characterizes aging in dogs. This is caused by loss of the melanocytes that are associated with hair follicles. Furthermore, a reduction in the number of hair follicles per square inch of skin accompanies aging, as does slower hair growth and hair of smaller diameter.

Sensory Changes

Nerve receptors for pressure and touch may be decreased in the very old dog. There appears to be a small increase in intensity required by stimuli in order to cause pain when applied to skin. Changes of this sort in the aged may be confused with changes in threshold that accompany the use of many medications that are analgesic or that affect perception.

Changes in Vitamin D Metabolism

The important role of the skin in production of active vitamin D has been discussed in the chapters Nutrition and Metabolism and The Endocrine System. In the skin, **7-dehydrocholesterol** is acted upon by ultraviolet light from the sun to form provitamin D_3, which is ultimately converted to the active form of vitamin D. Elderly animals may have limited exposure to sunlight. A deficiency of 7-dehydrocholesterol formation and a decrease in the size of the skin's vascular bed can contribute to vitamin D deficiency.

SKIN DISEASES

Pruritus

Elderly dogs often are taken to their veterinarians because of **pruritus**, an intense chronic itching. Visible lesions may or may not be clearly present. Pruritus is not a precise diagnosis because its causes are so varied and it is present as a symptom in so many skin diseases.

Failures of other organ functions may be associated with conditions affecting the skin. Chronic renal failure, several diseases of the liver, some blood conditions (including **anemia** and, occasionally, **lymphocytic leukemia**), **hypothyroidism**, and **diabetes mellitus** are among other diseases that are associated with pruritus.

The pruritus caused by **scabies** (**sarcoptic mange**) is notable for the intense itching it causes. Some of the drugs that may produce symptoms of pruritus are anabolic steroids, estrogens, progestins, phenothiazines, and erythromycin. Treatment should address the associated diseases, conditions, or medications. Local and systemic treatments are available, but many of these skin conditions are often resistant to localized treatment.

DERMATITIS

Dermatitis (inflammation of the skin) is a condition characterized initially by itching (pruritus), but it progresses to edema and reddening of the skin and, later, to exudation and crusting. Causes of primary dermatitis include contact with caustic chemicals, burns, abrasions, and allergic agents. It is important to determine and treat the primary condition, while providing symptomatic treatment for the skin. Secondary infection by bacteria, fungi, or parasites may be present. (When infection is primary, the skin condition is usually given its own descriptive name.)

The hair around lesions may be clipped for cleanliness and for ease in applying ointments and soaks. Corticosteroid-containing ointments are helpful, but they are not curative. Because dogs are likely to lick off surface medicines, oral corticosteroids may be required, but only after the veterinarian has determined that no infection will be made worse by the immune inhibition that may result.

Seborrhea is a condition that has two forms. A dry, flaky, and scaly type is secondary to other diseases such as mange, allergic dermatitis, or hormone imbalances. The other type is considered primary, although the cause is unknown. Cocker Spaniels and English Springer Spaniels are the breeds most affected.

In primary seborrhea, the skin is oily or greasy because of excess **sebum**, the secretion of sebaceous glands. Your veterinarian must distinguish the skin lesions from others that are related to mange, ringworm, and hormone-caused skin conditions. It is possible to control symptoms of seborrhea. Special shampoos, creams, and ointments will help. Secondary infection of the irritated skin must be avoided.

ACANTHOSIS

Acanthosis nigrans is a skin disease complex of dogs, frequently Dachshunds. The skin is thickened, darkly pigmented, and often has thorny growths at the sites of lesions. The diseased skin may first be noticed in the soft skin of the "armpit" or the thigh-abdomen junction. As it advances, hair loss occurs and lesions develop on other parts of the body, e.g., the undersurfaces of legs, flanks, flaps of ears, and anal areas. Hypothyroidism sometimes accompanies acanthosis, which is relieved when the thyroid condition is treated. In general, however, the cause of acanthosis is not understood. Cure is not likely, even with the current ability to treat endocrine deficiencies, but control is often possible.

IMMUNE-RELATED SKIN DISEASES

Older dogs, particularly, suffer from the uncomfortable, but uncommon, skin lesions of **bullous pemphigoid**, **pemphigus foliaceus**, **pemphigus vegetans**, and **pemphigus vulgaris**. They are caused by autoimmune attacks against intercellular materials that hold skin cells together. These skin conditions are discussed in detail in the chapter The Protective Role of the Immune System.

Food allergies, acute or chronic, may occur in dogs of any age. The symptoms are sometimes solely or primarily gastrointestinal. However, skin symptoms are common. Acanthosislike symptoms may be evident, and hypothyroidism or dermatitis from parasites (fleas, mites, etc.) must be ruled out. The skin condition caused by allergy to flea saliva or feces often persists after the fleas have been killed. When a food allergy seems likely, some type of elimination diet or a specific test with suspected foods is helpful. Brief use of corti-

176

costeroids will reduce symptoms, but appropriate modification of the diet provides long-term relief.

Allergic inhalant dermatitis is fairly common in dogs. A heredity tendency appears to exist. The offending **antigen** usually must be inhaled, but sometimes it is ingested or it penetrates the skin. Pollens, house dust, and molds are the most frequent allergens, as in humans. Dalmatians, Cairn Terriers, Scottish Terriers, West Highland White Terriers, and Wirehaired Fox Terriers are among the more susceptible breeds. Pruritus may lead to rubbing of the face and licking of the feet. Dry skin, scaling skin, earflap inflammation, and skin ulceration are signs of allergic dermatitis. Treatment consists of avoiding the offending substances. Sometimes, treatments to desensitize the dog may help, but only after skin testing has firmly established the antigens involved. As expected, corticosteroids will suppress the unwanted immune reaction, but concern about treatment-caused Cushing's syndrome (**hypercorticolism**) remains. Occasional use of antihistamines is claimed to help in some cases.

Drug allergies may produce skin symptoms and systemic effects. Vaccination reactions are the most common offenders because of the foreign material (e.g., egg protein) present in the vaccine. Penicillin is often an offender, among a number of other drugs. The specific skin reactions are varied. When mild, they may be self-limiting, but when more extreme, drug allergies may be life-threatening.

Allergic contact dermatitis, fairly uncommon in dogs, is initiated by contact with substances that combine with native proteins in the skin. The newly created protein molecules are foreign to the immune surveillance system, and an immune reaction develops against them. Flea collars are among the items that may cause this type of dermatitis. Symptoms, often where hair is thin or where surface contacts occur, include reddening and, later, hardening and pigmentation. Pruritus and exudation of the lesion may or may not be present. After ruling out other causes, treatment is directed toward the symptoms and avoidance of stimulating substances.

Systemic lupus erythematosus (SLE) has skin lesions that may be severe, although the disease may affect the whole body. The skin lesions include hair loss, reddening, and crusting. It is not a common disease of older dogs; it is more age-related in humans.

It is recognized that hair loss and skin inflammation are common in aging dogs. Conditions such as sarcoptic mange, caused by mites; **ringworm**, caused by fungi; **warts**, caused by viruses; and various reactions to fleas, mites, and lice may afflict older animals. However, it is not evident that these are age-related except that older dogs may be less able to defend against infection and infestation.

SKIN TUMORS AND CANCER

Tumors on or within the skin should always be respected, although many may prove to be benign. As a rule, benign tumors have a capsule around them and they grow slowly. Malignant growths characteristically grow rapidly and may spread (**metastasize**) to other tissues. The metastases are difficult to locate and quite difficult to treat or remove.

Benign tumors take many forms. Warts are caused by viruses; they need to be removed only if they are subject to injury or interfere with some function. **Lipomas** are encapsulated fat cells; they are rounded and soft, and they clearly are not firmly attached to surrounding tissue. They generally are not painful unless bruised. Although some lipomas are quite large, such growths ordinarily are not removed. **Sebaceous cysts** are derived from sebaceous glands. These cysts are also encapsulated, but their content is a cheesy substance rather than fat cells. They can become large and often become infected. Sebaceous cysts are reported to be more common in Kerry Blue Terriers, Schnauzers, and Spaniels. Only your veterinarian can determine whether any skin tumor is benign.

Modified skin glands in the area of the anus may give rise to benign **perianal gland tumors**, which must be differentiated from the occasional **adenocarcinomas** (cancers) that occur there. When these growths become ulcerated, infection and pain follow. These slow growths depend on the male sex hormone **testerone**. Castrated (neutered) animals have the advantage of being relatively free of them.

Mammary hyperplasia is characterized by a swelling of breast tissue, a tissue derived from embryonic skin glands (see the chapter The Reproductive System). This benign condition is most often seen in bitches that have not been bred recently, and spayed animals do not have mammary hyperplasia. Sometimes, an exudate can be expressed with pressure. Your veterinarian should observe the bitch in order to evaluate it and advise proper care.

About half of breast tumors are malignant. They appear as painless lumps, usually in older bitches. Your veterinarian should examine all mammary growths to determine if they are malignant because these cancers spread rapidly, especially to the lungs. If spread has not occurred, surgery is usually done to remove the breast tissue.

Malignant tumors of the skin generally invade adjacent tissue and grow rapidly. They may appear as ulcers that bleed. Some look like moles that suddenly begin to grow or bleed. Such lesions should be immediately seen by a veterinarian because the pigmented skin cancer **melanoma** has these characteristics. Melanoma rapidly metastasizes to other areas, making it quite life-threatening. Boston Terriers, Cocker Spaniels, and Scottish Terriers have been reported as common victims. Other cauliflowerlike, ulcerated growths may be **epidermoid carcinoma**. They itch and invite licking, resulting in hair loss in the area. These cancers, usually on the feet or legs, can be removed.

16

The Reproductive System: Age Changes and Consequences

$\mathbf{A}$LTHOUGH OLDER DOGS may sire or give birth to offspring, reproduction per se is not discussed here. Many good books on the subject are available and are more extensive than space will allow in this one.

MALE ANATOMY AND PHYSIOLOGY

The external male reproductive structures are the **penis** and the **scrotum**. The scrotum contains the **testes**. The penis is inside a penile sheath along the surface of the abdomen. The forward part of the sheath is called the **prepuce**. Secondary male characteristics include a somewhat larger body size than females of the same genetic type and a larger, stronger muscle mass. Although maleness is genetic, the expression of male characteristics is largely determined by tissue responses to male steroid hormones, particularly **testosterone**.

Sperm are produced in tubules of the testes. These tubules empty into a tubule at the upper part of each testis, the **epididymis**, which continues as a **vas**

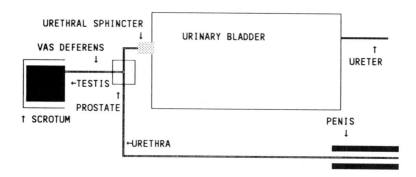

Male Urogenital System The urethra can be closed at the urinary bladder and thus used as a passage for sperm from both testes. A vas deferens from each testis joins and passes through the prostate gland, which adds its secretion to the sperm to form the seminal fluid. When urination occurs, the urine passes straight through the prostate gland. When enlargement of the prostate gland occurs, it may impede urine flow by pressing on the urethra, but in the dog, enlargement usually causes pressure on the rectum, which is nearby.

deferens. Each vas deferens follows a path over the top of the urinary bladder to the **prostate** gland, which surrounds the **urethra** where it leaves the **urinary bladder**. The right and left vas deferens join to form one common duct, which passes through the prostate gland and enters the urethra. The prostate gland has ducts of its own that enter the urethra in the same region. This system provides for the transport of sperm from the testes to the urethra, where they mix with secretions of the prostate gland to become the **semen** (the **ejaculate**).

Two spongy tissue masses are responsible for **erection** of the penis. They are cavernous bodies, making up a large part of the penile shaft. Each cavernous body has a large artery with branches that supply blood to infiltrate the spongy tissue. Dilation of arterioles in this tissue allows it to fill with blood at arterial pressure. Each cavernous body inflates until its size becomes restricted by the connective tissue sheath that surrounds it. This inflation constitutes erection.

The dog's penis differs from the human's in two notable ways. Toward the base of the penis there is a special mass of erectile tissue, the **bulbus glandis**. During erection, it inflates with blood, becoming a large globular structure that enables the "tie" with the bitch's vagina. Another feature of the dog's penis is a bone, the **os penis**, that begins beneath the bulbus glandis and runs toward the tip of the penis.

Erection and ejaculation are mediated by nerves of the **autonomic nervous system**. **Parasympathetic** nerve activity causes the dilation of arterioles that cause erection. Conversely, the contractions that result in emission of the semen involve **sympathetic** nerve activation. Stimulation of receptors on the penis initiates spinal reflexes that result in erection; nerve receptors at the rear of the bulbus glandis participate in the emission of semen. Although these reflexes are primarily spinal reflexes, they are influenced to a great degree by the central nervous system, which may inhibit or reinforce them.

180

FEMALE ANATOMY AND PHYSIOLOGY

The female's external genitalia are integrated with internal structures. Additionally, the female's breasts (**mammary glands**) represent secondary sexual characteristics that are developed because of endocrinological influences.

The **labia** are fleshy pads at the outer area of the **vulva** (external female genitalia). Interestingly, the embryonic tissues that become the labia are the same tissues that are developed into the scrotum of the male. The labia surround the **vestibule**, which contains the opening of the **vagina** and the external opening of the urinary tract (**urethra**). The **clitoris** is located in the lower portion of the vestibule; it is a small erectile structure, a female equivalent of the penis.

The vagina is the "birth canal" and the tubular structure into which the penis is thrust during mating. The vagina is separated from the **uterus** by the **cervix**, a sort of guard zone to help prevent contamination of the uterus and **uterine horns** with foreign material and bacteria. Cells of the vaginal wall change under the influence of sex hormones. Your veterinarian can examine a few of these cells under the microscope and learn a great deal about the condition and status of a bitch's reproductive cycle.

Uterine horns, which contain the fetuses during pregnancy, are lined with a layer of cells called the **endometrium**. The blood supplies of fetuses are in close proximity with the blood vessels of the endometrium.

Fallopian tubes (uterine tubes) arise from the upper portion of each uterine horn and lead to the **ovaries**. Eggs that are shed from the ovaries are drawn into the Fallopian tubes; fertilization of ova by sperm takes place in the part of the tubes near the ovaries. Fertilized eggs move into the uterine horns several days later.

The breasts, or mammary glands, are modified skin glands. This tissue has the ability to react to estrogens, which promote growth and development; functional maturity of the breasts follows stimulation by **progesterone** during pregnancy. If males are given regular doses of hormones or drugs that have estrogen

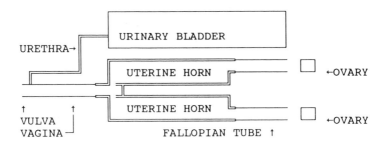

The Female Urogenital System   The two uterine horns that branch from the vagina and terminate in the vicinity of the ovaries are shown. Ova are fertilized in the Fallopian tubes by sperm that have been transported there from the vagina. The fetuses develop in the uterine horns, from which they are born. The urethra transports urine from the urinary bladder to the vulvar area.

181

activity, their breasts will develop as well. Glandular cells and milk ducts are the functional parts of mammary glands, and their effectiveness is not related to the size of the breasts.

REPRODUCTIVE ENDOCRINOLOGY

The fundamental aspects of endocrine control of the reproductive system are presented in the chapter The Endocrine System. The **hypothalamus**, in the brain, is the source of several releasing hormones that influence the cells of the **anterior pituitary gland**. Among them are the **gonadotropin releasing hormones** (GnRH). The two gonadotropic hormones produced by the anterior pituitary in response to GnRH are **follicle stimulating hormone** (FSH) and **luteinizing hormone** (LH). These received their names when early research showed the roles they played in female physiology. However, they are equally important and active in male physiology. The production of these hormones becomes significant at puberty in both sexes.

In mature bitches, FSH stimulates certain ovarian cells to develop into **follicles** (fluid-filled chambers), in each of which an egg matures. Cells that line a follicle are stimulated to produce estrogens by FSH. Cellular and endocrine responses are both part of FSH (and LH) action. When the follicle is properly developed, it ruptures in response to a surge of LH from the anterior pituitary gland. This is **ovulation**, the release of an egg.

The follicular cells that remain in the ovary respond to the influence of LH by undergoing further specialization to become **luteinized cells**, forming a **corpus luteum** (yellow body). This new tissue not only continues to produce estrogens in response to FSH, LH now causes it to synthesize the steroid progesterone.

In a similar fashion GnRH, FSH, and LH are functional in the male. However, the male cellular response is sperm production and the steroid hormone produced by the testes is testosterone. The male pattern is without the cyclic features that characterize bitches.

THE AGING REPRODUCTIVE SYSTEM

It is interesting that fundamental failure of the reproductive system, unlike other system failures, is not life-threatening to an individual. Various changes in the endocrine system have profound effects on the reproductive system's function. See the chapter The Endocrine System for more information on this overlap between system functions.

AGING CHANGES IN THE MALE DOG

Males of animals that have been studied undergo progressive endocrine and anatomical changes that alter quantitative and qualitative aspects of sexuality. Testosterone production seems to decline gradually in males but is present to some degree in the very old. Testicular cells from which sperm are produced remain active, producing somewhat reduced numbers of active sperm; old dogs that are physically capable of mating may still sire litters.

AGING CHANGES IN THE FEMALE DOG

Menopause is not evident in dogs, although some reproductive changes appear to accompany aging. Generally, litter size decreases in older animals, and poor health will certainly affect reproductive capabilities. Research observations apparently have not been made in dogs to understand all of the types of changes that occur in aging females.

DISEASES OF THE MALE REPRODUCTIVE SYSTEM

DISEASES OF THE PROSTATE GLAND

It has been claimed that about 60 percent of male dogs over eight years of age have **cystic prostate hyperplasia**, excessive growth of the prostate gland. However, many dogs do not show notable symptoms. An enlarged prostate may impede urine flow because of pressure on the urethra. In dogs, unlike humans, an enlarged prostate may press on the rectum and cause frequent, but ineffective, attempts to defecate, and constipation may result. Loss of weight and general condition may accompany marked prostatic hyperplasia. Chronic nephritis (see the chapter The Urinary System) is common in the same age group and must be differentiated from prostatic hyperplasia. It has also been noted that tumors of the Sertoli cells of the testes produce large amounts of estrogen, which causes a specific type of cell change in the prostate. Castration, by removing the source of testosterone, has proved quite useful in restricting prostatic growth.

Prostatitis (inflammation of the prostate gland) is more frequent in older dogs, and it is often associated with prostatic hyperplasia. Many different kinds of microorganisms may infect the prostate, and infection of the urinary tract is likely to spread to the prostate. Abscesses in the infected prostate are common. If they rupture, the microorganisms may enter the abdomen and produce life-threatening infection there. As in prostatic hyperplasia, symptoms of prostatitis may include pain, prostate enlargement, and urination and defecation difficulties. Blood may appear in the urine. Castration is a possible treatment, and antibiotics should be used to control the infection.

Various types of **prostatic cysts** have been described, sometimes associated with other prostatic diseases. Symptoms are like those in other conditions with prostatic enlargement. Some cysts may be small and cause relatively few problems; other large or numerous cysts may seriously affect the prostate and nearby tissues. Treatment includes removal or surgically draining the cysts.

Castration does not seem to be very helpful as an initial treatment, but it may be used to restrict further growth of cysts.

Cancers such as **adenocarcinoma** and **lymphosarcoma** may develop in the prostate gland. Signs may resemble other prostate disorders. However, because these cancers often metastasize (spread) to other tissues, symptoms may reflect the dysfunction of other malignant tissue. The enlargement or dysfunction of the other tissues may cause the symptoms that bring the dog to a veterinarian in the first place. Microscopic examination of affected tissues is needed for diagnosis. Castration and estrogen administration may help some. Otherwise, the prognosis is poor.

Tumors of the testes, prostatic enlargement, and prostatitis are prevented by early castration. Therefore, if a male dog is not important to a show career or breeding program, castration according to your veterinarian's recommendation should be seriously considered.

DISEASES OF THE PREPUCE AND PENIS

The prepuce of the dog provides an excellent environment for bacterial growth. Inflammation of the head of the penis and lining of the prepuce is called **balanoposthitis**. It is extremely common in a mild form and does not appear to cause problems. However, when the infection becomes severe, symptoms are more evident and may involve the whole animal. A discharge of pus, swelling and pain in the preputial area, fever, and generally apparent illness indicate a more serious condition. Your veterinarian can determine the infecting organisms and, thus, select the appropriate systemic antibiotic. An antibiotic ointment may be placed in the preputial space after it has been cleaned by flushing with a suitable antiseptic.

Infection in the prepuce may cause scar formation that prevents the penis from protruding through the opening (**phimosis**). Because this would make mating impossible, attempts to mate are accompanied by pain. When severe, phimosis may interfere with urination. Treatment may not be required, but surgery may be needed in other cases, a decision to be made by your veterinarian.

DISEASES OF THE TESTES AND EPIDIDYMIS

When the testes or tubules from it that store sperm cells are inflamed, it is called **orchitis** or **epididymitis**, respectively. Several bacteria or viruses, possibly spread from the urinary bladder or infected prostate gland, and trauma to the testicular area can cause acute inflammation of these tissues. See the discussion on **brucellosis** given below. Symptoms include swelling, pain, and fever, which may accompany rigid movement of the hind legs.

The acute condition may progress to a chronic form, and autoimmune problems may develop (see the chapter The Protective Role of the Immune System). Chronic orchitis or epididymitis also may be associated with cancer. Difficulty in determining the cause of the chronic condition makes treatment difficult. Also, if the affected animal is a valuable stud dog, retaining fertility may eliminate the option of castration, which would remove the inflamed tissue. Even when antibiotics and immunosuppressive drugs are used, fertility may still be lost.

Several types of cancer of the testes are seen. Undescended testes have a predisposition for developing cancer. Complete castration or removal of the involved testis are the treatments usually chosen. If cancer of the Sertoli cells occurs, the female hormone estrogen may be produced and feminization and anemia may develop. Of course, early castration would have prevented any of the cancers.

In dogs, the term **impotence** fits the broad definition of inability to perform the sexual act. Just as in humans, psychological bases are important. Dogs that have had negative experiences (punishment, aggressive bitches) or very limited association with other dogs may be reluctant to mate. On the other hand, sufficient testosterone, the male steroid hormone, is required to establish sexual drive. **Castration** (removal of the testes), of course, removes the source of testosterone. Tumors of the testes may produce estrogen, the female's sexual hormone, which will counteract any testosterone that is present. Estrogen may cause feminine characteristics such as breast development, changes in muscle structure, and attractiveness to other males.

DISEASES OF THE FEMALE REPRODUCTIVE SYSTEM

INFECTION AND INFLAMMATION

Pyometra is a unique condition of the endometrium in the uterus. For pyometra to occur, the endometrium's growth is first promoted by a high level of the hormone progesterone, normally needed to maintain pregnancy. However, in conditions that lead to pyometra, progesterone levels remain high following ovulation even when pregnancy does not occur. This results in growth and accumulation of endometrial secretions and, coincidentally, a suppression of the muscles of the uterus. A somewhat stagnant situation exists. This is an unfortunate invitation for bacteria from the vagina to infect the endometrium.

The other female sex hormone, estrogen, enhances the effects of progesterone. The use of large doses of estrogen to prevent unwanted pregnancy during the period following ovulation may substantially increase the risk of pyometra. A bloody vaginal discharge or a discharge with pus may be evident in some individuals. In others, the cervixes remain closed, discharge is not seen, and they are often quite ill before symptoms are noticed. Symptoms include frequent urination and thirst, lethargy, loss of appetite, diarrhea, and vomiting. The treatment that is most effective is **spaying** (removal of the ovaries and uterus).

If an attempt to preserve the breeding potential of the bitch is to be made, broad-spectrum antibiotics are given, fluid and electrolyte balance is maintained, and one of the **prostaglandins** ($PGF_{2\alpha}$) may be administered. The latter will cause relaxation of the cervix while promoting contraction of the uterine muscles. This helps expel the infected uterine material. If surgery is done in time, the prognosis is good. It may also be good in some of those that are medically treated. Your veterinarian's evaluation is important in determining the course of therapy and subsequent management.

Endometritis (inflammation of the endometrium) resembles pyometra except the enlargement of the uterus with accumulated material is less evident. Also, a complex involvement of hormones is not associated with endometritis.

Neither endometritis nor pyometra can occur if there is no uterus. Thus, if the bitch is not an important part of a breeding program or will not be shown in dog shows, *early spaying is highly recommended*. The dog's health is protected from these maladies, and the cost will ultimately be far less than treatment if these and other reproductive problems develop. Also, the absolute birth control is of value to most owners.

Vaginitis (inflammation of the vagina) is usually caused by bacterial infection. Cancer or other growths of the vaginal wall, infections in the urinary tract, and the administration of steroid preparations that have male hormone effects may be associated with vaginitis. The most common sign of vaginitis is a discharge, which may vary in character. Male dogs may be attracted by the odor of the discharge. This condition is not usually accompanied by systemic illness, which helps differentiate it from pyometra. Antibiotics and antiseptic vaginal douches are the usual treatments.

The uterus may become infected (**acute metritis**), especially after whelping. After delivery, a somewhat bloody vaginal discharge is usual for up to six weeks. However, if metritis is present, the discharge will have pus in it and a foul-smelling odor. The bitch will show symptoms of general illness and other signs with which your veterinarian is familiar. Antibiotics, supportive care, and injection of a prostaglandin or oxytocin are common treatments. Either of these injections cause the uterus to contract and expel infected uterine contents. Additionally, the ovaries and uterus may be removed at an appropriate time.

Mastitis is an inflammation of the breasts that may occur during the first six weeks following whelping. It may involve small or large areas, and it is not always accompanied with infection. Firm nodules, local warmth, and sensitivity to touch or pressure characterize the first symptoms. If systemic illness is present, there will be fever, loss of appetite, and changed appearance and behavior. Your veterinarian will choose antibiotics, taking into account that some may be passed on to the puppies through the milk. Further care is complex and based on many factors that should be appraised by a veterinarian.

Other Diseases of Female Sexual Tissues

Noncancerous growths of the vaginal lining (vaginal mucosa) is called **vaginal hyperplasia**. A tissue mass may protrude from the vulva, cause urinary difficulties, and, of course, impair mating. The mass will increase in size just before and during estrus and decrease in size during other times. This is caused by its sensitivity to the female hormones present. Your veterinarian will use a tissue sample to differentiate this growth from possible cancer.

Ovarian cysts are associated with production of large amounts of estrogen for a longer time than is usual for an estrous period. The vulva will likely remain enlarged because of high estrogen, as during a regular estrous period. Because of the hormone levels, acceptance of males may continue. These episodes are often variable and are not life-threatening. Your veterinarian can help manage the problem. If breeding is desired, it can often be arranged with veterinary help.

Cancer in Females

Bitches have fewer tumors of the reproductive tissue than males, and many tumors in females are benign. However, it has been reported that 10 to 15 percent of ovarian tumors are malignant, and the frequency is greatest in older bitches.

When tumors appear in the mammary gland (breast tissue), they are frequently **adenocarcinomas** (gland tissue cancer). It is estimated that 35 to 50 percent of a bitch's mammary gland lumps may be cancerous. It is the most common cancer in dogs except for those seen in the skin. This is interesting because the breast tissue is actually modified embryonic sweat gland tissue; the topic might as well have been discussed in the previous chapter on the skin. The only symptom usually seen by an owner is the lump or swelling in the breast. Your veterinarian may use biopsy (tissue sampling), X-ray, and other findings to evaluate the condition. Surgical removal of the growth, along with spaying, is a common treatment. If cancer spread is likely, chemotherapy may be used. If the growth is localized, its removal may provide a good outcome.

DISORDERS OF MALES AND FEMALES

If the bacterium *Brucella canis* infects the epididymis, testes, or scrotum, the dog often licks the scrotum excessively. The prostate may also harbor the organism. The infection is called **brucellosis**, and infected dogs often become permanently sterile. When a bitch has brucellosis, spontaneous abortion in the last trimester of pregnancy occurs. Sometimes there are earlier fetal deaths with resorption or stillborn puppies. Brucellosis may be spread to humans. Some veterinarians may recommend **euthanasia** ("putting to sleep") of infected animals because it is so infective and hard to control. No vaccine exists, and treatment is not as effective as desired.

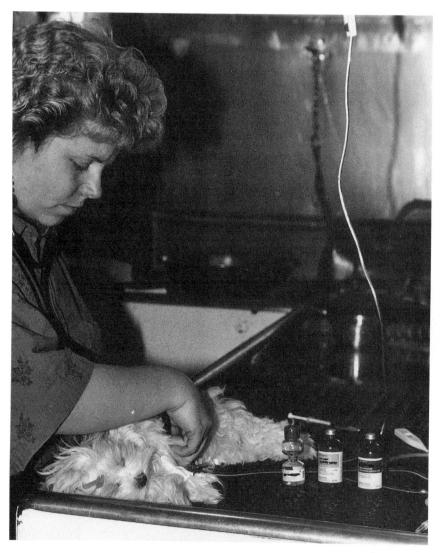

This veterinarian is using intravenous drug therapy on this dog to speed entry into the vascular system.

17

Drugs, Anesthesia, and Surgery in the Aging Dog

MODERN VETERINARY MEDICINE and the pharmaceutical sciences have made available an amazing array of drugs, anesthetics, and surgical and diagnostic techniques to benefit the older dog with health problems. Your veterinarian is constantly receiving information about new developments that may have important benefits to your older dog.

An annual physical examination for the older dog is vital to detect medical problems before they become severe. Your veterinarian may recommend examination of the blood cells (**hematology**) and **blood chemistry** (measurement of the quantity of many blood constituents, such as cholesterol, sodium, several enzymes) tests to provide added assurance that all is normal.

When an acute or a chronic disease is detected, medical management of the condition may require either surgical intervention or drug therapy. This chapter provides you with information to more fully understand the impact of surgery and/or drug therapy on your older dog.

DRUG THERAPY IN THE AGED DOG

Whether or not a specific drug will be both effective and safe depends upon many factors. Obviously, your veterinarian's instructions regarding the correct dose and the appropriate dosing duration must be followed carefully. Too low a dose or too long between doses will limit effectiveness. Too great a dose, given too frequently, will increase the risk of drug toxicity.

The correct dosage of a drug for a specific indication or disease, given at appropriate intervals, can be effective only if the proper concentration of the drug reaches specific tissues or cells that are the target. Drug disposition is divided into four stages: **absorption**, **distribution**, **metabolism**, and **excretion**, each of which is critical for effective and safe drug therapy.

Unless the target end point is within the digestive tract, when a drug is given orally, absorption must occur from the lumen of the stomach or intestine into the blood vessels associated with the digestive tract. The rate at which absorption occurs is influenced by many factors including the drug itself. Some sustained-release preparations are specifically manufactured to prolong absorption and thus reduce the frequency of dosing. The presence or absence of food in the digestive tract, and gastric and intestinal pH also play a part.

Although normal aging causes some changes in the digestive tract, these changes are not major factors in changing the rate of drug absorption. However, an owner should be constantly alert to problems within the digestive tract, such as vomiting or diarrhea, which may significantly decrease the amount of drug available for absorption.

Intravenous, intramuscular, and subcutaneous drug administrations are much less frequent than the oral route. These routes have a more rapid entry into the vascular system and more quickly attain therapeutic levels of a drug in the blood plasma.

The **distribution** of a drug occurs via the blood. Prior to reaching the general circulation, a drug absorbed from the digestive tract must first pass through the liver. Many drugs undergo important transformations in the liver. Depending on the presence of the necessary enzymes, the rate at which these reactions in the liver occur can have important consequences on the amount and rate at which a drug reaches the general circulation.

Distribution also includes the process of the drug leaving the blood vessels and entering the fluid between the cells and the cells themselves. The rate at which this occurs will depend on the nature of the drug. Those that are fat-soluble (**lipophilic**) will be able to pass more easily through the endothelium of capillary walls and other cell membranes, especially the body's fat cells. Compounds which are water soluble remain in the plasma for longer periods.

In both the older dog and older humans, there is a relatively increased amount of total body fat and a decreased amount of muscle and other lean tissue mass. Therefore, in the older dog carrying excessive weight, *body fat may serve as a drug reservoir that slows the rate drugs become available at target sites*. It was mentioned earlier that many drugs undergo metabolic changes in the liver. **Metabolism** is an important step in the process by which drugs are transformed into active or inactive metabolites prior to excretion from the body in either urine or bile.

The effect of aging on renal function has been discussed previously (see the chapter The Urinary System) and it was pointed out that degrees of renal failure are common in aging dogs. This is of special consequence during drug therapy because many drugs are eliminated from the body through the kidneys. Obviously, if drug elimination is impaired, repeated dosing may lead to toxic drug levels.

Only your veterinarian can evaluate how to modify drug doses in the older dog with renal impairment. In some cases, the effective dose will be lower than that for a younger animal. In other cases, standard doses will be used but with less frequent administration to allow for adequate but prolonged renal elimination.

ANESTHETICS AND PAIN CONTROL

Pain is a complex perception. Humans may experience pain under one set of conditions, but then at another time find the same stimulus not as painful. Pain may be exaggerated if stress is present. Some dogs, such as certain hounds, appear to tolerate considerable injury. By comparison, much lower stimuli may invoke pain in other breeds or individuals. This type of variation may be based on neurophysiological detection and transmission of stimuli, or may relate to central nervous system (CNS) processing of nerve impulses upon arrival at the brain.

Humans must attempt to understand what causes pain and painful responses in their dogs by using their own experiences. It must also be recognized that human perceptions of pain may be greatly influenced by emotional stresses that are difficult to apply to dogs. For example, it is unlikely that a hysterectomy in a dog will elicit emotional stress or concern about the animal's subsequent role in the human family. A dog may be up and about soon after major surgery, while a human may be more cautious about returning to regular activities. It is difficult to determine all of the factors that take part in a complex pattern of reactions to potential or actual pain.

Anesthetics are drugs that impair the brain's ability to perceive the environment, including feeling or sensation. They have made it possible for surgical procedures to repair injuries or correct anatomical errors. In addition to causing unconsciousness, anesthetics at proper doses usually make the patient immobile. Of course, if too great an amount is given, even respiratory muscles may be inhibited, creating a medical emergency.

Some dogs (e.g., Afghan Hounds, Collies, Greyhounds, Great Pyrenees, and Whippets) do not tolerate many anesthetics as well as other breeds. However, the choices among these drugs is great, and your veterinarian will be able to select an appropriate anesthetic for a procedure and for your dog's age.

Variations in effects of anesthetics and other drugs make some better for one purpose than another. **Barbiturates** are anesthetics that quickly produce unconsciousness, but, at proper doses, allow respiratory and some other reflexes to remain. **Analgesics**, such as morphine and codeine, are noted for their ability to deaden pain while allowing continued, although modified, awareness. Some of the newer anesthetics (e.g., halothane) and analgesics (e.g., fentanyl) are especially compatible with vital functions such as respiration, heart rate, and blood pressure. Anesthetics and analgesics generally have **sedative** (anxiety allaying) effects, but other drugs (e.g., **tranquilizers**) are especially useful in this respect. Some tranquilizers (e.g., diazepam or acetylpromazine) are used as preanesthetics. Depending on individual properties, they reduce anxiety, relax muscles, and reduce the amount of anesthetic subsequently needed. Atropine sulfate is often given before surgery to reduce saliva and mucus secretion and help keep the airway clear. Appropriate routes of administration vary with the chemical nature of the anesthetic; water-soluble barbiturates are usually given by injection, while halothane, a gas, is inhaled. Ether and nitrous oxide are two other gases with anesthetic properties.

Most injected anesthetics are longer-acting than most inhaled anesthetics. Long surgical procedures may favor long-acting anesthetics; short-acting ones allow quick recovery when its administration is stopped. Of considerable importance is the fact that some animal species respond differently to a given anesthetic. **Ketamine**, a newer injectable anesthetic, is often used to anesthetize dogs because it produces sedation to deep anesthesia depending on the dose administered, and it has a wide margin of safety (its lethal dose is much higher than its useful dose). **Peridural** (spinal) administration of agents to block pain sensations below the site of injection can be done in dogs, but it is not frequently used.

Anesthetics may be classified as general, in which all awareness is deadened, or local, in which specific areas are treated to block local sensations. Procaine and drugs derived from it are commonly used to produce anesthesia in local areas. In general, there is less risk to the health of a dog if local anesthesia is sufficient for a procedure.

Inflammation is associated with pain and anti-inflammatory drugs reduce pain, especially chronic pain. Some **corticosteroids** (e.g., hydrocortisone, prednisolone) are quite effective in suppressing inflammation, as are certain **nonsteroid compounds** (e.g., aspirin, phenylbutazone). **Narcosis** is a state in which sensation and awareness is numbed; morphine is a **narcotic**. **Tranquilizers** act on the brain and alter its ability to evaluate incoming sensations.

Anesthetic and analgesic drugs are removed from the body in several ways. Those that are inhaled are usually dispelled by the lungs, although some of the material may enter pathways in the liver or be lost by the kidneys. Ether has lost favor as an anesthetic because of its undesirable effects on the liver, as well as its flammability. Injected drugs are usually changed in the liver to some other form, rendering them nonanesthetic and, also, suitable for excretion. Liver and kidney diseases, relatively common in older dogs, may seriously compromise your veterinarian's choice of anesthetic. Furthermore, some of these drugs may lower blood pressure, which warrants caution in the elderly dog.

It has become common practice to use combinations of these substances in order to keep any one from overburdening the body's systems for handling them.

Also, **preanesthetics** are commonly used to reduce the anxiety of the dog and to reduce the amount of anesthetic needed to accomplish effective anesthesia. Some tranquilizers are good preanesthetics.

Anesthetics and related agents produce their effects in various ways. Aspirin, an anti-inflammatory drug, acts as an analgesic because it blocks an enzyme needed to synthesize certain **prostaglandins** (see the chapters The Endocrine System and the Blood and Body Fluids). These prostaglandins are involved in the production of inflammation, pain, and fever. Opium and its relatives act on the synapses between neurons, making it difficult for nerve transmission to take place. The volatile anesthetics halothane, ether, and nitrous oxide appear to act on selected brain areas to inhibit synapses there. Certain tranquilizers interfere with specific **neurotransmitters** of the brain so that information is not as effectively integrated and perceived as it should be.

The wide variation in the sizes of dogs because of age or breed makes it difficult to determine appropriate doses for all drugs. *Although body weight is commonly used, it should be used with caution.* This becomes more serious when the dog's metabolism has been altered by age-related changes. Rarely, drugs may not be effectively absorbed because of intestinal malfunction, and an old dog's blood may fail to reach a proper level for the substance. On the other hand, a drug may remain at high concentration for a longer time than usual because of failing liver metabolism and kidney function.

The dose and size relationship is often best resolved by associating the drug dose with the dog's **metabolic rate** (the rate of oxygen consumption). However, body weight does not precisely estimate a dog's metabolism. Considering that some breeds are well over fifteen times the weight of the smallest, quite an error of scaling might occur if weight alone is used.

In fact, it has been shown that the surface area of an animal is much more closely related to its metabolic rate than is its weight. Measurements have shown that smaller animals also have higher heart rates, respiratory rates, and, frequently, body temperature. If the goal is to have the anesthetic reach a certain level in the blood, body weight is an appropriate reference. The blood volume is about the same proportion of the total body weight in most normal dogs. If an anesthetic becomes concentrated in the brain, the relative sizes of the brains should be the factor considered in comparing doses for large versus small animals. Ultimately, your veterinarian must know the way in which any anesthetic is metabolized, whether it is concentrated in some tissue and its effect on activities such as respiration or liver function, and a number of other considerations.

SURGERY IN THE OLDER DOG

The stress of a hospital stay, anesthesia, and surgery may precipitate organ failure in older dogs. The most serious and likely consequences occur when the cardiovascular, respiratory, and kidney functions are affected. Older dogs may already have poor control of blood pressure, weakened contractions of the heart, and a tendency toward abnormal heart rhythms. Anesthesia and some surgical manipulations may aggravate any of these conditions. The respiratory muscles are weaker, nervous system control of respiration is less precise, and the lung's elastic recoil is reduced in older dogs. Measures should be taken to offset these problems when they exist. Otherwise, gas exchange may not provide adequate oxygen, and a failure to rid the body of carbon dioxide could easily lead to **acidosis** in the blood. Age-related changes in the kidneys may already have limited their ability to regulate the blood's pH and the blood volume. Reduced filtration and transport mechanisms make it difficult for the kidneys to excrete toxic metabolic products. Good liver function is also needed to handle many anesthetic by-products.

Surgery

It is not appropriate for this book to discuss surgical procedures in detail. However, the following paragraphs are meant to provide insight by brief examples. The choice of surgery on dogs with endocrine problems (see the chapter The Endocrine System) will help illustrate the rational thinking your veterinarian will bring to the treatment of your dog.

If a dog has **diabetes**, special attention is given whenever surgery is contemplated. Diabetics on insulin should have their current status evaluated and stabilized. The acid-base balance and water balance in these dogs are critical factors, as well as blood sugar levels. In general, most preanesthetics and anesthetics can be safely used in diabetic dogs. If surgery lasts longer than an hour, the veterinarian is likely to measure blood glucose at intervals. After surgery, very careful blood sugar control is required for effective wound healing.

Sometimes, tumors of the pancreas may involve the insulin-producing cells. Excess insulin causes a very low blood sugar. Removal of such tumors may be very challenging because damage of other parts of the pancreas will cause loss of other pancreatic functions. Most pancreatic tumors are malignant and may have already metastasized to other tissues. Your veterinarian will spend time stabilizing the dog's carbohydrate metabolism well before anesthesia and surgery. Often the extent of the tumor is not known until it is viewed during surgery. Relief of symptoms and life extension may occur in over half of all cases.

Dogs with **adrenocortical** (hormone) **insufficiency** are much more sensitive to the stress of surgery. Ordinarily, the production of corticosteroid hormones will increase severalfold during surgery; this is a normal response. Supplemental administration of corticosteroids to dogs with adrenocortical insufficiency may be carefully given to compensate for a dog's inability to respond appropriately. A proper blood level of corticosteroids is necessary to prevent low blood pressure and shock from collapse of the circulatory system. Your veterinarian will know which of the glucocorticosteroids to use in these circumstances.

On the other hand, **hyperadrenocorticism** (excess corticosteroid production) is seen in middle-aged and older dogs. It may be necessary to surgically remove one or both adrenal glands. Dogs with adrenal tumors and other causes of hyperadrenocorticism often have other health problems including high blood sugar, high blood pressure, electrolyte imbalances, skin lesions, and muscle wasting. Thus, the stress of anesthesia and surgery is a greater threat to the well-being of these dogs than it would be otherwise. Such dogs must be carefully monitored throughout anesthesia and surgery. Certain anesthetics, known to your veterinarian, are preferred in these cases. Because removal of the adrenal glands removes the source of corticosteroids, there will be a marked drop in these hormones following the surgery. Prompt administration of these hormones in proper doses may be required both during and after surgery.

In the later part of the 1980s, organ transplants were carried out by veterinarians. Many successful kidney transplants have been done in some veterinary medical centers. As in human medicine, immunosuppressive drugs such as cyclosporin and azathioprine have helped make the procedures effective. The ability to transplant pancreatic tissue to diabetic dogs is in the research phase.

A veterinarian's knowledge and care in selecting appropriate patients, choosing optimal anesthetics, and exercising skill in surgery are important to the outcome of surgery. However, knowledge of canine physiology is indispensable. It is required to make good judgments in managing an older dog's homeostatic state before, during, and after surgery; thus, it may be the most important element of all.

18

The Last Days

THIS RELATIVELY BRIEF CHAPTER will offer useful insights into the dynamics that surround a dog's final stage of life. It is hoped that it can be ultimately accepted as just that—a stage of life as respectable as all other stages since the beginning.

It may be useful to remember that no evidence exists to show that a dog is able to contemplate death the same way a human does. However, as normal functions slip beyond an ability to sustain life, dogs do clearly recognize their limitations and their dependency. Indeed, their apparent trust and need of support, while saddening, is also endearing.

When the special senses of hearing and sight deprive an older dog of its familiar environment, it may be easily startled by an unexpected touch—but how appreciated it is when the source is recognized. An elderly dog's reduced thirst drive, appetite, and ability to eat makes it vulnerable to thoughtlessness or carelessness. The fact that it rests and sleeps a great deal may make an owner overlook its need for physical contact, grooming, and examination for growths or lesions that may have developed.

A great deal of study of the human/animal bond has taken place during the past decade or so. Evidence exists that the first dogs were domesticated about 12,000 years ago, placing them, with horses and cats, in a special relationship to humans. There is reason to believe that remarkable genetic selection has occurred to make dogs unique in their ability to accommodate a life close to humans. Thus, it is not surprising that humans themselves feel the intensity of the bond that forms.

Recent surveys show that persons in our culture almost universally make photographs of their dogs, often including them in family portraits. Most individuals acknowledge that they talk to their dogs—and not just to give commands. Nearly all dog owners feel that they can sense their dog's mood and that the reverse is true. Less universal, but common, evidences of dog/owner relationships include celebrating a dog's birthday, taking it on trips as a travel companion, and allowing it complete sharing of the owner's living quarters. These indicate that the bonding is substantial and, in effect, gives the dog an integrated position of family membership. Consequently, the death of a dog would be expected to initiate the same kind of responses in an owner or family that the loss of any human member would invoke.

One feature of the dog/human bond relates to the perpetual child status of a dog. It is unlikely that a dog will be expected to "grow up" and assume progressively greater responsibilities. In fact, it is probable that the childlike role is a treasured part of a dog's relationship to the people close to it. Another feature of the relationship comes to the fore when a dog dies. Although public expressions of grief are encouraged when a human member of the family is lost, our culture is less willing to accept profound reactions of grief when the loss is the family's pet. However, substantial research indicates that surviving humans do suffer as though a human/human bond has been broken.

The same stages of bereavement are experienced as those following the death of a loved human: (1) denial of the death, accompanied by varying degrees of mental confusion; (2) anger that the death has happened, derived to some degree from the threat of facing the finality; (3) variable and vague guilt because of a sense that some responsibility might not have been met; (4) depression, with loss of pleasure responses and with low self-worth; and (5) resolution, in which there is sadness and the dog is missed, but with a progressive return to a satisfying life pattern.

When the death is sudden, perhaps violent, the denial phase may be quite prominent. If death follows chronic illness, guilt and a sense of failure may be a prominent experience. **Euthanasia** ("putting to sleep") may be the hardest death to accommodate. A lifetime of providing for a dog's health, development, and comfort seem reversed when death is elected. Many loving owners cannot entertain euthanasia and well-meaning friends should not make their suffering greater. Others see euthanasia as a gentle gift to end the dog's suffering in spite of the emotional pain they experience. This certainly does not mean that they love their dog less. Whether or not to be present during euthanasia is a highly personal matter and should be given considerable thought, perhaps with the help of an experienced counselor.

Many veterinarians and veterinary clinics have made arrangements to provide professional counseling for those who are contemplating their beloved dog's death or have recently experienced the tragedy. These therapists are especially skilled and experienced; the service they supply should be seriously considered when help seems needed. They understand the elements of crisis management: (1) they help in understanding what has happened, (2) they evaluate the availability of support from other persons and pets and help locate interpersonal support when needed; and (3) they help the bereaved individual develop coping skills if they are lacking. Children may have an unusually difficult time when any pet dies. Individuals who live alone will suffer exceptional loneliness when their dog is no longer with them.

Veterinarians are able to give clients pamphlets that discuss the death of pets and provide the titles of several good books that should help deal with the loss of one's dog. When emotional balance has been sufficiently regained or is stable enough, a library can help locate a copy of *The Last Will and Testament of an Extremely Distinguished Dog* by Eugene O'Neill, a grand way to remember a loved companion.

The aftermath of death contains other considerations: (1) Is the pet to be cremated and what is to be done with the ashes? (2) Is it to be left with the veterinarian for respectful disposal? (3) Will it be placed in a pet cemetery or can it be buried at home? (4) Should an autopsy be conducted? A beloved dog can be memorialized by planting a tree in one of its favorite places, by a gift to a carefully chosen animal welfare organization, by putting a memorial plaque in some special place, or by publishing a suitable notice in a dog publication. The contemplation and carrying out of a memorial activity will have comforting effects.

In addition, what to do about the void that the dog's death has left is an issue. Each person must meet individual and well-thought-out needs. Care must be exercised if a well-meaning gift of another dog is offered. A period of adjustment is often needed so that a new dog will not be expected to fulfill another's role. It is only fair that a new dog be allowed to fill a niche of its own—and owners are less likely to be disappointed.

EUTHANASIA

Euthanasia is the term used for a purposefully administered, painless, anxiety-free death. With the general availability of veterinarians, it is only reasonable that owners will choose their help and advice. Indeed, it is often the uncomfortable duty of a veterinarian to inform a dog's owner that the condition of a pet is terminal and warrants consideration of euthanasia. You may learn from your own veterinarian the methods currently in use. The discussion that follows is general.

The American Veterinary Medical Association's Panel on Euthanasia issues a consensus report of the most expedient techniques available. As even newer methods become known, your veterinarian will learn of them by reading regular veterinary science publications. Additionally, the AVMA is active in educating veterinarians about the reactions and needs of bereaved humans.

A number of methods of euthanasia exist, and some are suitable only for certain animals. The methods that are best for dogs may include the reduction of anxiety prior to administration of a lethal agent. In some cases, the dog's personality and confidence in humans may make anxiety unlikely; whether the presence of a calm owner will help should be discussed with the veterinarian. Any method of euthanasia requires skilled veterinary personnel who can make the recommendations suitable for the specific circumstances.

Glossary

THIS GLOSSARY is arbitrarily limited, but it should be an aid in understanding many terms that are not familiar to lay readers. Also, definitions given are meant to serve the usage found in this book; other definitions of terms could be added but are not needed here.

acetylcholine (ACh)   A neurotransmitter molecule in somatic and parasympathetic neurons—acts between neurons and between neurons and their target cells. Acetylcholinesterase is an enzyme that inactivates acetylcholine.

action potential   The collapse and restoration of the electrical potential across nerve and muscle cell membranes, which is propagated along the membrane—the "impulse."

adenosine monophosphate (AMP)   A nucleotide with adenosine as its base and one attached phosphate group.

adenosine triphosphate (ATP)   A nucleotide with adenosine as its base and three attached phosphate groups, two of which are held by high-energy bonds that serve as the primary coupled energy source for all of the body's metabolism.

adrenal cortex   The outer layer (cortex) of the adrenal gland, it is the origin of corticosteroid hormones such as aldosterone and hydrocorticosterone.

adrenal medulla   The inner part (core) of the adrenal gland, it is the origin of hormones such as epinephrine (adrenaline) and norepinephrine (noradrenaline).

adrenocorticotropic hormone (ACTH)   A hormone of the anterior pituitary gland that stimulates production of steroid hormones by the adrenal cortex.

adrenocorticotropic releasing hormone (CRH)   A hormone produced by the hypothalamus that causes production of corticotropic hormone by the anterior pituitary gland.

albumin   Produced by the liver, it is the smallest, but most abundant, major plasma protein. It is important in osmotic regulation, as a nutritional protein reserve, and as a transport agent for other molecules.

aldosterone   A mineralocorticoid from the adrenal cortex, it is involved in electrolyte balance, such as promoting sodium conservation by the kidney.

allergy   An immune state or hypersensitivity to specific substances (allergens) that are responded to by release of tissue histamine, which results in various reactions in vascular, respiratory, and other smooth muscles.

alveolus (alveoli)   A lung air sac wherein gas exchange takes place.

amine   A molecule that contains an amine group ($-NH_3$).

amino acid   A molecule with a terminal carbon atom that has both an amine group ($-NH_3$) and the acid carboxyl group ($-COOH$) attached to it.

amyloid   A group of proteins that accumulate in small blood vessels, injuring them. The condition is called *amyloidosis*.

analgesic   Something, usually a drug, that relieves pain.

anaphylactic shock   A fall in blood pressure caused by the action of released histamine from mast cells in response to an immune reaction.

anemia   Literally means ''without blood''—a misleading interpretation. Refers to a condition in which the blood hemoglobin concentration is lower than normal without regard to the cause. For example, iron deficiency anemia and hemolytic anemia are two types caused, respectively, by lack of sufficient iron or fragile, easily destroyed blood cells.

angiotensin II   A potent peptide vasoconstrictor and stimulator of aldosterone production. It results from enzymatic (renin) conversion of the plasma protein angiotensinogen to angiotensin I, which in turn is the precursor that angiotensin converting enzyme (ACE) converts to angiotensin II.

antibody   A protein that has been specifically synthesized to bind to a foreign molecule (antigen). It is an agent of the immune system, produced by plasma cells (derived from B lymphocytes).

antidiuretic hormone (ADH)   It is produced by neurons of the hypothalamus, released at the posterior pituitary. It acts on the kidney to regulate water conservation. It is also called *vasopressin*.

antigen   A molecule to which the immune system responds by producing specific antibodies or specific cellular sensitivity.

antioxidant   As used here, a substance that becomes oxidized by accepting the transfer of hydrogen ions ($H+$), thus protecting some other substance that might be oxidized.

aorta   The body's largest systemic artery, it leaves the left ventricle and distributes branches to all of the body.

arteriole   A small arterial branch just preceding capillaries; the vascular element most responsive to nerve and chemical stimuli that affect changes in peripheral resistance to blood flow.

artery   Blood vessels especially able to tolerate pressure that carry blood away from the heart.

arthritis   A degenerative disease of bone joints.

ascites   Essentially, edema of the abdominal space, which enlarges because of accumulated fluid.

ATP   See **adenosine triphosphate.**

atrium   Either of the two upper heart chambers that receive returning blood from the body and lungs.

atrophy   To waste away or become smaller.

autoantibodies   Antibodies that react against certain of the body's own molecules, having been produced when the immune system failed to recognize these molecules as self. Sometimes the error is in the recognition mechanism; at other times slight alteration of the antigen molecules may have occurred.

autoimmune   An immune reaction against cells or substances of the self, caused by a failure of the immune system to distinguish between self and foreign material.

autonomic nervous system (ANS)   A specific motor portion of the nervous system that is generally involuntary and controls the visceral organs and part of the skin. It has two divisions, the sympathetic and the parasympathetic.

axon   The process of a neuron that conducts impulses away from the cell body.

basal ganglia   A specific group of neuron cell bodies (a ganglion) located deeply in each cerebral hemisphere.

basophil   A granular leukocyte (white blood cell) that has an affinity for basic dyes.

B cell lymphocytes   Can be transformed into cells called *plasma cells* that are able to respond to antigens by the production of specific antibodies to them.

benign   Not malignant, i.e., not cancer-causing.

bile   The fluid of the gallbladder. Formed in the liver, it contains bile salts, pigments, cholesterol, etc., and is emptied into the small intestine.

blood group   A category of red blood cells established by identifying a genetically determined antigen on the surface of the cells.

blood plasma   The cell-free portion of the blood; it contains water and all of the soluble material of blood.

blood platelet   A fragment from a bone marrow cell, the megakaryocyte, found in the blood. They participate in blood coagulation and blocking minor leaks in blood vessels.

blood serum   The fluid portion of whole blood following blood coagulation. It resembles blood plasma except for the modification caused by the chemical reactions of clotting (coagulation).

blood sugar   Glucose, a monosaccharide derived by the digestion of carbohydrates such as starch.

body fluids   The water and its solutes found in various body spaces, e.g., intravascular space, extracellular space, intracellular space, etc.

bone marrow   The cells, fat, and other material that fill the inner core of bones. The cells there give rise to the cells of the blood and immune system.

Bowman's capsule   A capsulelike chamber found in the kidneys that surrounds a tuft of capillaries (glomerular capillaries) and receives a protein-free, cell-free filtrate of the blood, which is subsequently processed into urine.

bradykinins   Polypeptides that are primarily vasodilators.

brain stem   The medulla oblongata, pons, and midbrain.

bronchi   The main air passages of the lungs. Bronchioles are smaller branches.

bundle of His   Named for an investigator named His, this modified cardiac tissue rapidly conducts an action potential from the atria to the ventricular muscle.

calorie   The amount of heat needed to raise the temperature of one gram of water by 1°C. In the field of nutrition, 1 C is one kilocalorie, one thousand calories.

cAMP   See **cyclic adenosine monophosphate**.

capillary   The smallest blood vessel, it has lost the characteristic muscle and connective tissue coating of arteries and is an endothelial tube, especially suitable for water and soluble exchange between blood and interstitial fluid.

carbohydrate   A class of compounds made of carbon, hydrogen, and oxygen, which serves as a primary source of energy in the biological system, as well as structural roles.

carcinogens   Agents that participate in the development of cancer.

cardiac   Refers to the heart. Cardiac muscle is heart muscle; cardiac output is the amount of blood pumped per minute.

castration   To remove the testes.

catabolism   The breakdown of molecules from complex to simpler forms.

cell membrane   The polarized lipoidal (fatty) surface surrounding cells. It serves many functions, such as protecting cell contents and providing means of transporting substances across it. It possesses molecules that identify cells immunologically, and possesses molecules to bind various substances in order to effect cell function.

central nervous system (CNS)   The brain and spinal cord.

cerebrospinal fluid   Found in the ventricles of the brain and associated with the meninges, it is produced by the choroid plexus.

cerebrum (cerebral)   Composed of the right and left hemispheres, this is the largest part of the brain and the portion serving the most advanced mental functions.

chemoreceptor   A nervous system receptor that is easily stimulated by specific chemicals or chemical reactions.

chromosomes   Molecules of DNA that contain the genes. Referred to as chromatin (colored) material. Sex chromosomes are one pair and somatic chromosomes are the remainder of chromosomes in a cell.

cilia   Hairlike projections from the surface of some cells that, by waving motion, may move the cells or may move the fluid about such cells.

collagen   Produced by connective tissue cells, a giant protein molecule that forms the matrix of bone and soft tissue throughout the body.

congestive heart failure   An inability of the heart to effectively pump out the blood received, resulting in pressure backed into the veins, especially the pulmonary veins, causing pulmonary edema to form.

cortex   The outer layer of an organ or structure.

corticosteroid   A steroid hormone produced by the adrenal cortex.

corticotropin (ACTH)   See **adrenocorticotropic hormone.**

cyclic adenosine monophosphate (cAMP)   A form of adenosine monophosphate that acts as a second messenger to initiate cellular activity following the cell's reaction with membrane-bound stimulants.

cytoplasm   The cellular components outside the cell's nucleus.

cytotoxic   An agent that will kill cells.

dendrites   The projections of a neuron that carry impulses toward the cell body.

deoxyribonucleic acid (DNA)   A nucleotide polymer (chain) containing the sugar ribose and a nucleotide base in each unit; it accommodates the coding of genetic information according to the sequences of the bases.

dermis   The deep layer of the skin, the layer below the outermost layer, the epidermis.

diabetes insipidus   A condition characterized by a diuresis of dilute urine as a result of a deficiency of antidiuretic hormone (ADH) and its effect of promoting water reabsorption by the kidney.

diabetes mellitus   Caused by a lack of insulin or a reduced sensitivity to it, this condition is characterized by high blood glucose levels and a spillover of glucose in the urine. It may be accompanied by other degenerative tissue changes.

diastole (diastolic)   The period in the heart cycle when the muscle is not contracting. Also, refers to the blood pressure present during the period of heart diastole.

diuretic   Any substance that promotes increased urine excretion. There are many types acting via various mechanisms.

DNA   See **deoxyribonucleic acid.**

duodenum (duodenal)   The first portion of the small intestine, immediately following the stomach.

edema   The accumulation of excess fluid (interstitial fluid) in the spaces between cells, having leaked from malfunctioning capillaries or accumulated from faulty drainage via the lymphatic channels.

elastin   A large, elastic protein produced by connective tissue cells found in most tissues.

electrocardiogram (ECG)   The record, also called EKG, of electrical activity that takes place because of the progression of the action potential throughout the heart and its repolarization.

electrolytes   Ions and ionized molecules that are able to conduct an electric current. Because of their abundance, they play an important role as particles in the osmotic forces across the membranes of the cells.

embolus (emboli) A blood clot in the bloodstream that has broken away from its origin.

endocrine gland A hormone-producing gland that secretes directly into the blood via neighboring capillaries.

endogenous Refers to something that arises within the body.

endothelium Epithelial tissue that lines blood vessels and the heart chambers.

enzyme One of many specific protein molecules that have the property of catalyzing equally specific chemical reactions.

eosinophil A leukocyte that has an affinity for the acidic dye eosin.

epidermis The outermost layer of skin.

erythropoiesis The process of red blood cell (erythrocyte) production in the bone marrow.

esophagus The tubular part of the digestive tract that leads from the pharynx to the stomach.

essential amino acid Any required nutritional amino acid that must be ingested because the body has no way to synthesize it.

estrous That stage in the reproductive cycle when the bitch is sexually attractive to males.

euthanasia Intentionally putting an animal to death to save it from suffering.

fatty acid Organic compounds composed of carbon chains, hydrogen atoms, and an acidic carboxyl group ($-COOH$) on a terminal carbon.

fibrin An insoluble protein that collects in a network to form a blood clot following its conversion from the soluble fibrinogen by an enzyme, thrombin.

follicle A fluid-filled chamber, e.g., an ovarian follicle.

follicle stimulating hormone (FSH) A gonadotropic hormone from the anterior pituitary that stimulates steroid production by ovaries and testes; it participates in the production of ova and sperm.

free radical A highly reactive ion that contains unpaired electrons. Such ions are short-lived because they so easily react with other ions or molecules, usually oxidizing them.

gallbladder A bladder attached to the liver, from which it receives bile and stores it until emptying into the small intestine.

ganglia Groups or special collections of nerve cell bodies.

gastric Refers to the stomach or its functions.

gastrin A hormone that is produced by certain stomach cells and stimulates other stomach cells to produce hydrochloric acid and pepsinogen (pepsin precursor)

gates Cell membrane structures that act as selective channels for specific substances.

genes A particular sequence of nucleotides in DNA that represent the sequence of amino acids in a protein that a cell can synthesize.

gerontologist The student of aging in all of its aspects.

glomerular filtration rate (GFR) A measurement of the volume of blood that is filtered through the glomeruli of the kidney in a minute.

glomerulonephritis Inflammation of the renal glomeruli with failure of normal kidney function.

glomerulus (glomeruli) A tuft of capillaries surrounded by Bowman's capsule, from which an ultrafiltrate of the blood is formed.

glucocorticoids Steroid hormones from the adrenal cortex that have many functions, including effects on glucose, fat, and protein metabolism. They also suppress immune reactions and inflammation.

gluconeogenesis The formation of glucose from other than carbohydrate, especially from amino acids.

glycoprotein A molecule in which glucose is complexed with a protein molecule.

growth factors Any of a number of substances that induce cell multiplication, usually produced and active locally, unlike hormones.

growth hormone A hormone of the anterior pituitary gland that promotes bone and soft tissue growth; it influences fat, carbohydrate, and protein metabolism throughout life.

heartworm A parasitic worm; the adults reside in or near the right side of the heart.

helper T cells/helper T lymphocytes A subpopulation of lymphocyte T cells that are involved in promoting antibody production by B cells.

heme The iron-containing portion of hemoglobin.

hemoglobin The oxygen-carrying molecule of red blood cells; it is composed of heme and a protein (globin) moiety.

hemorrhage To lose blood following injury to blood vessels.

herbivores Animals that primarily consume plant material as food.

homeostasis The dynamic constancy of the body for which almost all of the bodily functions are responsible.

hormone A molecule that is produced by an endocrine gland, secreted into the bloodstream, and carried to target cells where specific reactions are invoked.

humoral immunity Those immune reactions that involve production, distribution, and action of antibodies.

hydro- A prefix indicating water.

hyper- A prefix meaning higher or more than.

hypertension Excessive blood pressure.

hypertrophy Growth of an organ caused by increased cell size.

hypo- A prefix meaning lower or less than.

hypoglycemia Blood glucose below the normal range.

hypothalamic Refers to the hypothalamus of the brain, a portion of the forebrain with many functions, including regulation of the pituitary gland and influences on the autonomic nervous center.

hypothyroidism A condition in which thyroid function is deficient.

hypoxia A low blood oxygen concentration.

ileum The last of the three parts of the small intestine.

immunoglobulins Various proteins within the globulin classification that have been synthesized to function as antibodies.

impulse The progressive depolarization wave along a nerve or muscle membrane and the progression of the process from one cell to another.

incontinence Inability to control defecation or urination.

insulin A polypeptide hormone of the beta cells of the pancreas that affects cell membranes so that glucose enters more easily and fat and amino acid metabolism is effected. Without insulin, blood sugar is high, is not available for metabolism, and spills over into the urine—the condition is called *Type I diabetes.*

interstitial space That space outside the blood vessels that surrounds body cells.

inulin A polysaccharide of fructose that is filtered but not secreted or reabsorbed by renal tubules, making it suitable to measure the glomerular filtration rate (GFR).

in vitro Occurring outside the body, as in a test tube.

in vivo Occurring within the body.

islets of Langerhans Clusters of pancreatic cells that produce insulin and glucagon.

jejunum The second, or middle, segment of the small intestine.

keratin The insoluble protein of skin, hair, and nails.

ketone bodies Acetone, acetoacetic acid, and beta-hydroxybutyric, which are derived from metabolism of fatty acids by the liver. When present in excess, the condition ketosis exists.

killer T cells/killer T lymphocytes Immune system cells of the adaptive immune system that particularly attack virus-infected cells.

Krebs cycle The metabolic pathway by which decarboxylation and oxidation reactions occur as energy is ultimately derived and CO_2 is produced when food molecules are degraded.

lactose A disaccharide of glucose and galactose, called *milk sugar*, it is digested by the enzyme lactase.

large intestine Consists of the cecum and colon, ending in the rectum and anal canal.

larynx Located at the upper end of the trachea, it contains the vocal cords; commonly called the voice box or "Adam's apple."

lens Behind the pupil of the eye, the lens is a transparent, refractive protein that changes shape to vary the focus of objects viewed.

lesion An area of injury.

leukocyte Numerous kinds of white blood cells with a variety of functions, among them immune response, fighting infection, etc.

lipid A fat molecule.

lipofuscin A fat-containing pigment that accumulates in aging cells, causing brown areas when deposited in the skin.

lipoidal Referring to fatty nature.

lipoprotein A complex formed by a lipid and a protein molecule.

lumen The space within a tubular structure in which substances (e.g., blood, food, etc.) move.

luteinizing hormone (LH)   A gonadotropic hormone from the anterior pituitary that stimulates steroid (progesterone) production by ovaries, and participates in the production of ova and sperm.

lymph   The solution of material found in the lymphatic system, essentially that found in the interstitial space.

lymphatic system   A plasmalike fluid (lymph) is derived from the interstitial fluid and travels through the lymphatic ducts and lymph nodes to great veins near the heart.

lymphocyte   One of several small white blood cells; they are characterized by lack of cytoplasmic granules.

lymphokines   A group of chemical agents that provide information exchange (stimuli) among cells involved in immune functions.

medulla   The central area of an organ.

medulla oblongata   A portion of the brain stem at the top of the spinal cord.

melanin   The dark pigment of skin and hair, it is derived from the melanin-producing melanocytes of the epidermal layer of skin.

messenger RNA (mRNA)   The complementarily coded nucleotide strands that are synthesized in association with DNA (transcription), and which serve as templates for protein synthesis (translation).

metabolic rate   The level of metabolism as reflected by the amount of oxygen used per minute.

metabolism   All of the chemical processes of living cells.

mitosis   The usual process of cell division that results in two daughter cells essentially the same as the original.

monocyte   A relatively large, phagocytic white blood cell.

monosaccharide   A simple sugar molecule, such as glucose, fructose, and galactose.

motor   A term reflecting action. The motor area of the brain sends action potentials via motor neurons to motor units of muscles to initiate contraction.

mucosa   A mucous membrane that lines tracts or cavities that communicate with the outside of the body.

nasal gland   A structure in a dog's nose that can secrete large amounts of water, the evaporation of which cools the blood flowing through that tissue, helping cool the body.

natural killer cell (NK)   An immune cell of the innate immune system that especially attacks virus-infected cells.

nematode   One of a class of roundworms, some of which are parasitic.

nephron   The functioning unit of the kidney, it consists of a glomerular tuft of capillaries, Bowman's capsule, a system of tubules, and a peritubular network of capillaries.

neuron   The highly differentiated nerve cell; consists of dendrites, cell body, axon, and axonal endings.

neurotransmitter   Chemical agents that are released by the axon endings of one neuron and react with receptors on the dendrites or cell bodies of other neurons, helping propagate the action potential from one to another neuron.

neutrophil   The most abundant white blood cell, it is a phagocyte distinguished by its shape and staining characteristics.

node of Ranvier   A bare area between myelin investments of axons.

norepinephrine   A catecholamine related to epinephrine originating from the adrenal medulla and also serving as a neurotransmitter at some nerve synapses.

nucleus (nuclei)   The core structure within cells that contains DNA. Otherwise, a group of cells with like function, e.g., in the central nervous system.

oncogene   A gene that controls production of growth factors that participate in the development of cancerous cells.

organ   A structure of two or more tissues that performs a specific function.

organelle   Microscopic, functional structures within a cell.

organism   An individual living creature.

osmosis (osmotic)   The water-holding property of a substance that cannot pass through a membrane that is otherwise permeable to water.

osmotic pressure/force   It is expressed as mm of Hg (mercury) and measured by allowing an equilibrium to occur after a solute-containing solution is placed on one side of a water-only permeable membrane and water alone is on the other side. At equilibrium, the solute-containing water will have risen in its compartment (drawing water from the other) to a height that represents the pressure it can generate.

osteoblast   A bone-forming cell.

osteoclast   A cell that erodes and reabsorbs bone.

ovum (ova)   The mature egg.

pancreas   A mixed gland (endocrine and exocrine) that produces the hormones insulin and glucagon; it also produces and delivers to the small intestine sodium bicarbonate and enzymes that digest fat, carbohydrate, and protein.

para-aminohippuric acid (PAH)   A substance used to measure renal blood flow because it is almost completely eliminated from the body by filtration and secretion as it traverses the kidney.

parasympathetic   A division of the autonomic nervous system, it acts to suppress some activity and excite others.

parathyroids   Small glands embedded in the thyroid gland that produce parathyroid hormone (PTH), which causes bone resorption and raises blood calcium levels.

pepsin   The stomach's protein-digesting enzyme.

pH   Refers to the hydrogen ion concentration of a solution; it indicates the degree to which it is acidic or basic. When the pH is 7.0 it is neutral; above 7.0 indicates a basic solution, while below 7.0 is progressively more acid.

pheromone   A substance produced by one animal that has physiological effects on another animal of the same species. Its effects resemble those of hormones, although they are airborne.

phospholipids A triacylglyceride (fat) molecule in which a phosphate group has replaced one of its fatty acids.

physiology The science concerned with the mechanisms of life processes.

pineal gland A small gland located near the third ventricle, it originated as nervous tissue but primarily retains connection to the brain via a blood supply.

pituitary gland A small gland consisting of anterior and posterior parts that lies below the hypothalamus, with which it has intimate neuronal and vascular connections. It is the source of several hormones and the point of release of others.

plasma The fluid portion of blood, in which the cells are suspended and which contains the plasma proteins, electrolytes, etc.

platelets/blood platelets Cytoplasmic fragments of megakaryocytes of the bone marrow, they participate in hemostasis and blood coagulation.

polypeptide A chain of amino acids; when large, it is called a *protein molecule*.

polysaccharide A chain (polymer) of monosaccharides. Examples are starch and glycogen.

polyunsaturated Fatty acids that have a number of sites at which carbon atoms share double bonds with one another, thereby not having all of the possible sites occupied with hydrogen atoms.

pons That part of the brain just above the medulla oblongata.

posterior pituitary That lobe (the neurohypophysis) of the pituitary that receives axons bringing oxytocin and antidiuretic hormone from cells in the hypothalamus.

preanesthetic An agent, often a tranquilizer, given before anesthesia to reduce the amount of anesthetic required or to enhance its effect.

prepuce The foreskin of the penis.

progesterone The steroid hormone of the female upon which continued and healthy pregnancy depends.

prolactin A hormone of the anterior pituitary gland that stimulates milk production (lactation) and may participate in regulating gonadal function.

promoter A term used to indicate something that affects a stage in cancer development following the action of an initiator, which makes the initial alteration in cellular DNA.

prostaglandin Certain fatty acid-derived hormones that act locally, affecting smooth muscle contraction, acid secretion in the stomach, inflammation, and pain.

prostate gland Surrounding the urethra where it exits the urinary bladder, it adds an alkaline solution to the ejaculate (semen); its enlargement by benign or cancerous growth may impede urine flow and cause pressure on the rectum.

proto-oncogene A gene that, with suitable alteration, can become an oncogene, a gene that participates in cancer cell behavior.

pulmonary Refers to the lungs and their function.

receptor   A specialized structure that acts as a transducer and converts one form of energy (chemical, light, mechanical, etc.) into an action potential that can be transmitted to the central nervous system.

red blood cells (RBC)   Cells produced in the bone marrow and released into the blood. They cannot multiply directly because they have no nucleus; they are red because they contain the oxygen-carrying pigment hemoglobin.

releasing hormones   Specific hormones produced by the hypothalamus that act on the anterior pituitary, causing it to produce its relevant hormones.

renal   Refers to the kidney and its functions.

retina   The layer at the rear of the eye that contains the photoreceptors that respond to light.

RNA (ribonucleic acid)   Any of several nucleic acids, including mRNA, tRNA, and rRNA.

rod   A non-color-sensitive photoreceptor of the eye that is especially suited to perception of light at low levels.

scent glands   Modified sweat glands that produce distinctive substances, the odor of which identifies the species and, often, the individual. Dogs have such glands in their anal sacs.

Schwann cell   A cell that invests peripheral nerve axons with a myelin sheath.

second messenger   A chemical agent released or activated when a cell responds to a reaction with a hormone, neurotransmitter, or other chemical influence that brings about a more specific cellular reaction, such as enzyme activity or membrane changes.

semen   The fluids and substances of the ejaculate in males, it contains spermatozoa and originates in the testes and prostate gland.

semilunar valve   One-way half-moon-shaped valves that guard the ventricular exits to the pulmonary artery and aorta.

serum   See **blood serum.**

shock   See **anaphylactic shock.**

solute   Material that is dissolved in a solvent, such as water.

solvent   A substance, e.g., water, capable of dissolving solutes.

somatic   Refers to the parts of the body that are not visceral.

spayed   To have had the uterus removed. Commonly, the ovaries are also removed.

sphincter   A ring of muscle that controls flow through a tubular structure, such as from the stomach to the intestine or from the urinary bladder to the urethra.

spleen   An organ that plays a major role in removing and destroying old or damaged red blood cells from the circulation and helping recycle the iron and protein from them.

stem cells   Relatively primitive cells that give rise to other cells. For example, bone marrow cells are the origin of blood cells, and germinal cells of the gonads give rise to ova or sperm.

steroid   Compounds made of three carbon rings on the pattern of cholesterol; the steroid hormones are all examples.

stress As used, stress refers to profound reactions of physiological systems to stimuli that exceed their ability to maintain the usual homeostasis. Not to be confused with emotional distress unless it is profound.

stroke Loss of effective blood flow to some part of the brain caused by rupture of a blood vessel or a blood vessel's occlusion by a blood clot.

suppressor T cells Those T cells that have the ability to suppress the activity of other lymphocytes.

sympathetic A division of the autonomic nervous system, it acts to suppress some activity and excite others, although it is frequently excitatory.

synapse The juncture of one neuron's process with that of another, where impulse transmission is accommodated by production of a chemical neurotransmitter.

systole The period of the heart cycle during which the myocardium is contracted.

systolic pressure The blood pressure reached as the result of ejection of a stroke volume.

T cell/T lymphocyte Lymphocytes that participate in cell-mediated immunity, in which cells directly react with foreign or targeted cells or material.

testosterone A steroid of the androgen class that is produced primarily by the testes, but also the adrenal cortex in small amounts; it causes development of the features known as masculine and causes sex drive.

thorax The chest; thoracic refers to thorax-related parts and function.

thymus gland A lymphoid organ in which lymphocytes receive immune-related stimuli and undergo alteration in their functional roles, and in which hormonelike substances (thymosins) are produced.

tissue A group of similar cells that are collected together and function collectively.

trachea The airway from the larynx until it branches into bronchi in the lungs.

trypsin A proteolytic enzyme in the pancreatic juice.

unsaturated fatty acid Refers to a fatty acid carbon chain that has some portions lacking all of the hydrogen atoms that could be bound.

urea When amine groups are removed from amino acids or other sources, the liver makes urea from them; urea is then excreted as a waste product by the kidney.

uremia Retention in the blood of urea and other products of protein catabolism because of inadequate kidney function.

ureter A duct that leads urine from a kidney to the urinary bladder.

urethra A duct that leads urine from the urinary bladder to the outside of the body.

uterus/uterine horns Commonly called the *womb*, the uterus is largely smooth muscle and connective tissue, able to grow and accommodate a developing fetus during pregnancy.

vagina The tubular structure that connects the uterus to the outside of the body at the genital vestibule. Commonly known as the birth canal, it accommodates the penis of the male during sexual contact and receives the semen from ejaculation.

vein A less muscular blood vessel than an artery, the vein conveys blood back toward the heart under low pressure.

ventricles Chambers, e.g., ventricles of the heart or in the brain.

venule A small blood vessel that receives capillary blood and delivers it to a vein.

virus (viral) An infectious agent composed of DNA-like or RNA-like chains of nucleotides, along with other genetic codes and proteins, including a protein outer coat.

vulva The female's external genitalia.

white blood cells (WBC) See **leukocyte**.

X-rays Energy waves, having some of the characteristics of light rays, but able to alter molecules such as DNA and form free radical ions from water molecules.

Index

Anaplasia, 13
Ancylostoma caninum, 73
Androgens, 81, 213
Anemia, 76, 85, 87, 88, 100, 102, 135, 136,
    140–42, 156–58, 175, 185
  iron deficiency, 88
  macrocytic, 85
  pernicious, 85
Anesthesia, 116, 192–95
Anesthetics, 189, 191, 192, 194, 195
Anger, 198
Angiotensin, 109
Angiotensin II, 114, 202
Ankylosing spondylitis, 168
Anorectal strictures, 77
Anorexia, 58
Anterior chamber of the eye, 40
Anterior cruciate ligament, 168
Anterior pituitary, 46, 48, 50–56, 81, 182
Antibiotic action of saliva, 63
Antibiotics, 35, 84, 117, 126, 129, 143, 148,
    150, 153–55, 183–85, 186
Antibodies, 80, 134, 136, 144, 149–50, 153,
    156, 157, 202
Antibody-mediated immunity, 153
Anticholinergic substances, 76, 192
Anticoagulants, 83, 133, 138
Antidiuretic hormone (ADH), 48, 52, 53, 62,
    100, 113, 114, 202
Antigens, 136, 148–50, 151, 153–55, 158,
    170, 177, 202
Antihistamines, 125, 131, 177
Anti-inflammatory drugs, 143, 168, 192
Antioxidant, 87, 202
Antiseptic, 184, 186
Antithrombins, 143
Anti-thyroid drugs, 56
Anus, 63, 64, 69, 76, 77, 149, 171, 178
Anxiety, 30, 192, 199
Aorta, 94, 111, 202
  pressure in, 95
Apnea, 36
Apneustic center, 123
Apocrine glands, 59
Appetite, 30, 85, 87, 105, 143, 185, 186, 197
  hypothalamus and, 61
Aqueous humor, 40, 42
Arachnoid membrane of brain, 35
Arginine vasopressin, 53
Arrector pili muscles, 173
Arrhythmias of the heart, 105
Arterial pressure, 95, 180
  See also Blood pressure
Arteries, 94–97, 99, 100, 104, 107, 111, 143,
    172, 180, 203
Arterioles, 94, 202
Arthritis, 26, 54, 55, 156, 158, 203
Artificial insemination, 137
Ascarid nematodes, 73
Ascites, 104, 106, 141, 203
Ascorbic acid, 85
Aspiration, 130
Aspirin, 87, 112, 138, 143, 167, 192, 193
  prostaglandins and, 62

Assimilation, 2, 80
Association functions of brain, 27
Asthma, 126, 127, 130, 149
Astrocytes, 35
Ataxia, 37, 85
Atherosclerosis, 104
ATP. See Adenosine triphosphate
Atria, 93–97, 105, 107, 203
Atrial natriuretic factor, 114
Atrio-ventricular (A-V) node, 96
Atrio-ventricular (A-V) valves, 94
Atrophic gastritis, 70
Atrophy, 203
Atropine, 72, 192
Audition, 28, 30, 35, 39, 41, 43, 44, 197
Auditory association area, 28
Auditory centers in brain, 44
Auditory sensory area, 28
Autoantibodies, 153, 154, 156, 158, 203
Autoimmunity, 25, 82, 147, 164, 174, 176,
    184
  activity, 154
  blood and lymphatic system, 156
  concept of, 152
  endocrine system, 157
  eye, 42
  hemolytic anemia (AIHA), 142, 156, 202
  multiple sclerosis, 25
  muscle cell nucleus, 156
  musculoskeletal system, 155
  myasthenia gravis, 25
  myelin, 37
  skin, 158
  thyroiditis, 55, 157
  vaccines, live virus, 56
Autointoxication, 76
Autonomic motor nerves, 33
Autonomic nervous system (ANS), 4, 30, 31,
    33, 34, 95, 99, 180, 203
  check-and-balance system, 4
  gastrointestinal control, 67
  heart rate, 98
  injury, 38
  salivary glands, 65, 69
Autopsy, 199
Aversion, 22, 30
AVMA Panel on Euthanasia, 199
A-V node, 97, 105
A-V valves, 94–96, 104
Awareness, 33, 192
Axons, 20, 21, 25, 203
  regeneration, 36
  terminals, 18, 20, 22–24, 27
Azathioprine, 195

Bacteremia, 117
Bactericidal, 172
Bactericidal properties of saliva, 65
Bad breath, 72
Balanoposthitis, 184
Barbiturates, 191, 192
Basal energy requirement (BER), 91
Basal ganglia, 30, 203
Basement membrane of the epidermis, 158

217

Basophils, 134, 142, 146, 148, 149, 154, 203
Basset Hounds, 128
B cells (B lymphocytes), 135, 140, 148, 149,
    151
Beagles, 25, 36, 77, 91, 143, 168
Behavior, 29, 30, 37, 51, 54, 186
Belladonna, 72
Benign prostatic hyperplasia (BPH), 118, 203
Beriberi, 84
Beta-carotene, 84
Beta-endorphin, 23
Bicarbonate, 49, 139, 141
Bile, 61, 67, 68, 70, 74–76, 82, 112, 136,
    158, 198, 203
    See also Bilirubin
Bilirubin, 70, 136
Binocular vision, 40
Biological clocks, 5
Biotin, 85
Birth canal, 181
Birth control, 186
Bitch in heat, 41
Bitter taste, 65
Bladders, 30, 33, 111, 115, 116
Bloat, 74
Blood and body fluids, 2, 4, 93, 100, 129,
    133, 138, 141, 149, 203
    chemistry, 109, 112, 125, 189, 194
    hemoglobin, 102
    plasma, 35, 138, 139, 141, 203
    plasma protein, 68, 76, 80, 100, 101, 109,
        128, 130, 134, 141, 143, 202, 211
    sugar (glucose), 5, 60, 91, 194, 195, 203
    temperature, 98
    viscosity, 100
Blood-brain barrier, 20, 35
Blood cells
    red blood cells. See Erythrocyte
    white. See Leukocytes
Blood coagulation, 75, 76, 83, 86, 98, 99,
    129, 132, 134, 135, 137, 139, 143, 203
    intravascular, 34, 100, 129, 138, 143, 144,
        212
Blood flow in
    brain, 34, 163
    intestinal mucosa, 70
    nephrons, 111
    pulmonary, 119
Blood group, 133, 136, 153, 203
    incompatibility, 133
Blood platelets, 133–35, 137–40, 143, 144,
    148, 157, 158, 203, 211
Blood pressure, 30, 34, 48, 53, 57, 86, 99–
    102, 106, 128, 141, 154, 192–95
Blood transfusions, 106, 133, 141, 144, 157
Blood vessels, 2, 4, 33, 37, 48, 93, 103, 120,
    171, 172, 203
    See also Arteries; Arterioles; Capillaries;
    Veins; Venules
Blood volume, 53, 86, 100, 102, 105, 106,
    121, 139, 193, 194
Body cooling, 121
Body fat, 30, 190
Body fluids, 106, 117, 129, 133, 139, 141

Body temperature, 30, 102, 123–25, 172–74,
    193
Body weight, 7, 90, 105, 193
Bolus, 65, 66
Bone, 50, 54, 86–88, 161, 164–66
Bone marrow, 16, 88, 114, 134, 135, 140–44,
    148, 155, 157, 165, 204
Bordetella, 131
Boston Terriers, 57, 76, 77, 126, 178
Botulinum toxin, 24
Bowel control, 38, 76
Bowman's capsule, 113, 204
Boxers, 14, 54, 57, 126, 166
Bradycardia, 105
Bradycephalic airway syndrome, 126
Brain, 2, 28, 29, 31, 34–36, 38, 81, 106,
    162, 163, 182, 191–93, 204
Breasts, 149, 169, 178, 181, 182, 185–87
Breathing. See Pulmonary; Respiratory system
Breeding program, 186
Breeds, 3, 38, 40, 43, 44, 55, 57, 65, 73, 74,
    77, 103, 104, 115, 127, 131, 144, 155,
    168, 191, 193
    life spans of, 6, 7
Breed standards, 65
Bronchi, 105, 120, 121, 123, 124, 130, 154,
    204
Bronchial asthma, 127
Bronchioles, 48, 120, 121
Bronchitis, 130, 131
Bronchodilators, 131
Brucellosis, 184, 187
Bulbus glandis, 180
Bulldogs, 40, 126
Bullous pemphigoid, 158, 176
Bundle of His, 96, 204
Burns, 142, 175

Caffeine, 89
Cairn Terriers, 177
Calcification, 84, 87, 125
Calcitonin, 55, 58, 114, 165
Calcium, 50, 79, 80, 86, 88–90, 97, 139,
    161–64
    absorption, 68, 70, 84, 88, 165, 166
    absorption and dietary fiber, 89
    balance, 88
    corneal, 43
    excretion, 88
    heart valve deposits, 103
    hyperexcitability and, 86, 97
    kidney transport, 89
    loss, 89, 165
    metabolism, 58, 88, 89
    transport protein, 88
Calculus, 71
Caloric needs, 91, 124, 204
Caloric restriction, 6, 89, 155
Cancer, 9, 10, 13–16, 76, 77, 87, 90, 91,
    142, 152, 154
Cancers, types, 77
    adenocarcinoma, 13
    carcinoma, 13
    chondrosarcoma, 13

228

Nerve growth factor, 20, 81
Nerve impulse, 20, 21, 23
Nerve membrane, 21
Nerve paralysis, facial, 26
Nerve receptors
  cough reflex, 123
  drugs, mind altering, 23
  nipple area, 52
  osmo receptors, 55, 100
  penile erection, 180
  sensory, 32, 33
  skin, 173, 174
  special senses, 39, 40, 41, 42, 44
  taste, 165
  types of, 22, 204, 209, 212
Nerves, 2, 19, 22, 23, 36, 171
Nervous control
  control of respiration, 194
  heart, 95
  skin, 173, 174
  urination, 111
Nervous system, 3
  autoimmune, 25
  categories of function, 27
  stress, 3
  virus, 25
Neuritic plaques, 37
Neuroendocrinology, 30, 45
Neuroglia, 20, 35
Neurological complications of distemper, 129
Neurological symptoms, intervertebral disk
  disease, 168
Neuromodulators, 22, 23
Neuromuscular dysfunctions and swallowing,
  73
Neuromuscular transmitter, 164
Neuronal interconnections, 27
Neuronal plasticity, 36
Neurons, 9, 12, 18, 20, 52, 193, 209
  aging, 25
  cell body, 20, 28, 36
  chain of, 22
  communication mechanisms, 22
  connections, 22
  dendrites, 20
  malnutrition, 25
  medications, 25
  somatic motor neurons, 23
Neuropathy, 26
Neurophysiology, 30
Neuroreceptors, 123
Neurotoxin, snake venoms, 24
Neurotransmitter, 33, 36, 163, 164, 193
  acetylcholine, 23
  receptor binding, 22
Neurotransmitters, 22–25, 33, 156, 163, 164,
  201, 209, 210, 212, 213
Neutered, 178
Neutral fats, 82
Neutropenia, 142
Neutrophilia, 142
Neutrophils, 134, 142, 148, 210
NGF. See Nerve growth factors
Niacin, 85

Niacinamide, 85
Nicotinamide, 85
Nicotine, 85
Nicotinic acid, 85
Nictitating membrane, 38
Night blindness, 84
Night vision, 43
Nipples, 171
Nitrous oxide, 192, 193
NK cells. See Natural killer cell
Nocioreceptors, 22
Nodal rhythm of the heart, 105
Nodes of Ranvier, 22, 23, 210
Non-erosive polyarthritis, 156
Non-steroidal compounds, 192
Norepinephrine, 33, 48, 58, 98, 125, 210
Nose, 149, 154, 158, 159
  See also Nasal cavity
Nose breathing, 44
Nuclear membrane, 11
Nuclear sclerosis, 42
Nucleic acids, 85, 153
Nucleus, 11–13, 20, 148, 156, 205, 210, 212
Nutrients and exercise, 79
Nutrition, 2, 3, 90, 136, 159, 163
Nutritional anemia, 136
Nutrition and cancer, 90

Obesity, 82, 83, 90, 91, 131, 168
Occipital lobe, 29
Odor, 22, 65, 186
Ointments, 176
Old English Sheepdogs, 128
Olfaction, 29, 30, 39, 41, 44
Oligodendrocytes, 20
Oncogenes, 10, 14, 210
O'Neill, Eugene, 199
Opacities of the lens, 42, 84
Opiod. See Morphine
Opium, 193
Optic nerves, 40
Oral cavity, 121
Oral disease, 69
Oral mucosa, 158
Oral tumors, 72
Orchitis, 184, 185
Organelles, 11, 12, 210
Organ of Corti, 44
Organophosphates, 25
Organs, 2, 210
Organ transplants, 155, 195
Orthopedic surgery, 166
Osmoreceptors, 53, 100
Osmotic action
  electrolytes, 86
  forces, 141
  plasma proteins, 80, 100
  pressure, 21, 101, 139, 141, 210
Osmotic stress on red blood cells, 140
Os penis, 180
Ossicles, 41, 43
Osteitis, 166
Osteoarthritis, 88, 155, 167
Osteoblasts, 165, 166, 210

229

Plasma membrane, 10
Plasma proteins, 68, 80, 100, 101, 128, 134, 141
Plasma volume, 80, 139
Plasmin, 138
Platelet. *See* Blood platelets
Pleural effusion, 129
Pleural membranes, 120, 128
Pleural space, 128, 129
Pleurisy, 121
Pleuritis, 121, 129
Pluripotent stem cells, 134, 135, 148
Pneumonia, 72, 126, 129, 130
Pneumotaxic center, 123
Pneumothorax, 128, 129
Poisons, 7, 75, 87
  See also Toxins
Polarization (depolarization), 21–23, 86, 95, 97, 204, 205, 208
Pollens, 127, 154, 177
Polyarthritis, 156
Polymyositis, 156, 164
Polypeptides, 80, 211
Polysaccharides, 68, 154, 211
Polyunsaturated fatty acids, 84, 211
Pomeranians, 131
Pons, 29, 31, 123, 211
Poodles, 57, 60, 77, 131, 168
Positive feedback systems, 4
Posterior chamber of the eye, 40
Posterior cruciate ligament, 168
Posterior pituitary, 52, 53, 211
Posture, 163, 166
Potassium, 21, 86, 88, 97, 139, 163
  excretion, 25
  hypoexcitability, 86, 97
Potassium levels, heart action, 86, 106
Preanesthetics, 192–94, 211
Prednisolone, 192
Pregnancy, 50, 136, 145, 181, 185, 187
Prepuce, 179, 184, 211
Presbyesophagus, 69
Presbyopia, 42
Pressure in the ventricles, 95
Primary motor area, 28
Primary seborrhea, 176
Procaine, 192
Progesterone, 50, 53–55, 56, 114, 181, 182, 185, 211
Progestins, 175
Progressive retinal atrophy, 43
Prolactin (PRL), 51, 52, 55, 211
Prolactin inhibiting factor (PIF), 51
Propylthiouracil, 56
Prostacyclin, 138
Prostaglandins, 46, 61, 62, 82, 112, 123, 138, 173, 186, 193, 211
  aspirin and, 62
  blood pressure, effect on, 100
  fatty acids, 45
  molecular life span, 61
  source, 61
Prostate gland, 52, 116–18, 180, 183, 184, 187, 211

adenocarcinoma, 184
cancer, 118
cysts, 183
growth, 183
hyperplasia, 77, 117, 118, 180, 183, 184
lymphosarcoma, 184
pressure on rectal area, 76
Prostatitis, 116, 118, 183, 184
Protamine-zinc insulin, 60
Protein-free filtrate, 100
Proteins, 11, 20, 21, 24, 42, 51, 52, 55, 57, 68, 76, 80, 82, 84, 92, 100, 134, 143, 149, 151, 153, 154, 158, 161–63, 171, 172, 177, 202, 207, 211, 214
complexes, 80
deficiency, 80
diets and kidney disease, 81
digestion, 80
electrically charged, 21
energy yield, 82
excretion, 158
hormone influences, 81
intake, 80, 88, 163
malnutrition, cardiovascular shock, 106
metabolism, 80, 85
metabolism and cancer, 90
molecules, 80
muscle, 162
synthesis, 81
Proteins in blood coagulation. *See* Blood coagulation
Proto-oncogenes, 14, 211
Provitamin D_3, 175
Proximal convoluted tubule, 111
Pruritus, 175, 177
Pseudorabies, 20
PTH. *See* Parathyroid hormone
Ptyalism, 72
Puberty, 5, 31, 50, 152, 172, 182
Pug, 126
Pulmonary, 107
artery, 94
artery and dirofilaria, 107
blood flow, 96, 119
blood vessels, 130
capillary bed, 125
circulation, 94, 95
edema, 104, 120, 125, 130, 131
efficiency, 102
gas exchange, failure of, 104
inflammation, 127
obstructions, 130
system, 2, 119, 120, 122, 211
tuberculosis, 129
vein pressure, 104
ventilation, 102
  See also Respiratory system
Pulmonary thromboembolic (PTE) disease, 143
Pulse, blood pressure, 99
Punishment, 30
Pupil of the eye, 38, 40, 42
Puppies, 186
Pus, 184–86

cancer, 185
steroid hormones, 46
tumors, 184
undescended, 144
Testosterone, 50–53, 55, 56, 81, 117, 118,
    165, 178, 179, 182, 183, 185, 213
and muscle mass and strength, 81
Tetanus toxin, 20
Tetany, 86
Thalamus, 29–30, 52
Thiacetarsamide, 107
Thiamin, 84
Thiazide diuretics, 59
Thirst, 185, 197
Thoracic nerves, 32
Thoracic spinal cord, 37
Thorax, 100, 121, 123, 213
Thrombocytes. See Blood platelets
Thrombocytopenia, 143, 157
Thrombocytosis, 144
Thrombosis, 143
Thromboxane A, 138
Thrombus (thrombi), 143
Thymosins, 52, 61, 152
Thymus gland, 14, 46, 52, 61, 148, 151, 152,
    154, 155, 159, 213
involution, 152, 154, 155
Thyroglobulin, 153
Thyroid gland, 26, 46, 51–55, 58, 81, 176
Thyroid hormone, 38, 46, 51, 52, 87, 114,
    165, 172
metabolic effects, 55
production, 55, 165
protein synthesis, 55
thyroxine, 55, 81
types, 55
tyrosine, 46
Thyroiditis, 55
Thyroid stimulating hormone (TSH), 51, 53
Thyrotropin, 51, 53, 55
Thyrotropin releasing hormone (TRH), 48, 51
Tick paralysis, 20
Ticks, 142
Tidal volume, 122, 123
Tie with bitch, 180
Tissue culture, 15, 16
cells in, 10
contact inhibition and, 16
life span, 10
Tissue repair, 79, 81
Tissue transplantation, 147
Tissue-type plasminogen activator (t-PA), 138
T lymphocytes, suppressor, 14
Toenails, 169, 170, 172
Tongue, 42, 65, 66, 69, 72, 85, 123, 124
Tonsillitis, 127
Tonsils, 63, 152
Tooth loss, 69, 71
Torsion, 74
Touch, 65
Toxic drug levels, 191
Toxins, 73, 75, 149, 163, 194
Trachea, 66, 120, 121, 123, 124, 130, 149,
    213

Tracheobronchitis, 131
Tranquilizers, 30, 192, 193
Transferrin, 68
Transfusion, 106, 136, 141
See also Blood transfusion
Transplants, organ, 195
Transport systems
intestinal, 80
renal, 112
Trenchmouth, 72
Triacylglycerols (triglycerides), 68, 82
Tropic hormones, 53
Trypsin, 70, 213
Tryptophan, 85
Tuberculosis, 126, 129, 157
Tumors
brain, 20
pericardial space, 106
skin, 178
ureters, bladder and urethra, 118
Tympanic membrane, 41, 44
Type I diabetes, 60
Type II diabetes, 60, 91
Typhus, 75
Tyrosine, 46

Ulcerations, 141, 158, 178
Ultraviolet (UV) light, 42, 169, 170, 175
Unconsciousness, 31, 191
Undescended testes, 185
Urate uroliths, 115
Urea, 36, 80, 87, 116, 139, 141, 213
Uremia, 36, 116, 117, 213
Ureters, 110, 111, 113, 115, 116, 118, 213
Urethra, 111, 115–18, 180, 181, 213
Uric acid, 112, 115, 116, 141
Urinary
bladder, 31, 38, 111, 113, 115–18, 180,
    181, 184
incontinence, 117, 168
system, 109, 114, 167, 181, 183, 186
tract obstruction, 117
Urination, 33, 111, 116, 117, 180, 183–85
Urine, 75, 113, 158, 180, 190
blood in, 145
bloody, 118, 183
color, 136
pH, 115, 116
volume and diuretics, 101
Urokinase, 138
Urolithiasis, 115
Uroliths, 115, 116
Uterus, 33, 50, 52, 181, 185, 186, 213
endometrium, 185
horns (tubes), 181
muscles, 186
smooth muscle, 62

Vaccine, 73, 75, 131, 153, 177, 187
Vagina, 149, 180, 181, 185, 186, 213
Vaginitis, 186
Valves
atrio-ventricular (A-V), 94, 95
cusps, adhesions of, 103